Assessment Scales in Depression, Mania and Anxiety

Raymond W Lam, MD, FRCPC
Professor and Head, Division of Clinical Neuroscience
Department of Psychiatry, University of British Columbia
Vancouver, BC, Canada

Erin E. Michalak, PhD
Research Associate, Division of Clinical Neuroscience
Department of Psychiatry
University of British Columbia
Vancouver, BC, Canada

Richard P Swinson, MD, FRCPsych, FRCPC
Professor and Chair, Psychiatry & Behavioural Neurosciences
Morgan Firestone Chair in Psychiatry
McMaster University, Faculty of Health Sciences
Department of Psychiatry and Behavioural Neurosciences
Hamilton, Ontario, Canada

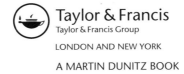

Taylor & Francis
Taylor & Francis Group

LONDON AND NEW YORK

A MARTIN DUNITZ BOOK

© 2005 Taylor & Francis, an imprint of the Taylor & Francis Group

First published in the United Kingdom in 2005
by Taylor & Francis, an imprint of the Taylor & Francis Group,
2 Park Square, Milton Park, Abingdon, Oxfordshire, OX14 4RN

Tel.:   +44 (0) 20 7017 6000
Fax.:   +44 (0) 20 7017 6699
E-mail: info@dunitz.co.uk
Website: http://www.dunitz.co.uk

A CIP record for this book is available from the British Library.

Library of Congress Cataloging-in-Publication Data

Data available on application

ISBN 1 84184 434 9

Distributed in North and South America by

Taylor & Francis
2000 NW Corporate Blvd
Boca Raton, FL 33431, USA

Within Continental USA
Tel.: 800 272 7737; Fax.: 800 374 3401
Outside Continental USA
Tel.: 561 994 0555; Fax.: 561 361 6018
E-mail: orders@crcpress.com

Distributed in the rest of the world by
Thomson Publishing Services
Cheriton House
North Way
Andover, Hampshire SP10 5BE, UK
Tel.: +44 (0)1264 332424
E-mail: salesorder.tandf@thomsonpublishingservices.co.uk

Composition by Scribe Design, Ashford, Kent, UK
Printed and bound in Italy by Printer Trento S.r.l.

Contents

5
Special Populations   167

Series preface

The use of assessment scales in psychiatry is becoming much more part of clinical practice. The availability and obvious utility of instruments combined with a pressing need to measure more precisely how we practise, may have served as stimuli for their increased use.

The success of *Assessment Scales in Old Age Psychiatry* was pleasing and it is very logical that a book outlining scales for the common disorders of depression and anxiety should be published. Drs Lam, Michalak, and Swinson are to be congratulated on producing such an excellent compendium. The layout and design is innovative and the description of the scales is comprehensive and clinically useful.

One of the stimuli for writing *Assessment Scales in Old Age Psychiatry* was that I was fed up trying to locate all the instruments from old photocopies of articles, which always seemed to get lost. *Assessment Scales in Depression, Mania and Anxiety* is a formidable contribution to the field and the text is a real must for practising psychiatrists. The book should also be useful to general practitioners, psychologists, researchers, students and other mental health workers. It does so much more than rid you of all those irritating pieces of paper and has the real potential to improve the care we provide to our patients.

Alistair Burns
Head, School of Psychiatry & Behavioural Sciences
Professor of Old Age Psychiatry
University Manchester
Wythenshawe Hospital
Manchester, UK

Introduction

The proper use of assessment scales can help improve the clinical care of patients with common, debilitating psychiatric conditions such as depressive and anxiety disorders. Assessment scales serve the same role as laboratory tests in other areas of medicine and have similar strengths and limitations. Assessment scales should not be used in isolation nor should they replace a clinical evaluation, just as one should not treat a laboratory result without considering the clinical status of the patient. Nothing can take the place of a comprehensive evaluation of a patient. However, an appropriate assessment scale can complement the clinical assessment and provide a convenient, short-hand method to track clinical progress.

This book was conceived to be a practical clinical resource for psychiatrists, family physicians, other mental health practitioners and for students in those disciplines. While there are several excellent books that give very detailed psychometric information about various assessment instruments, there are few that provide a user-friendly collection of rating scales for busy clinicians. This book strives to meet several objectives to serve this important clinical need. First, it provides a quick reference for clinicians to select an appropriate assessment scale to use for a specific clinical indication in patients with depressive, bipolar and anxiety disorders. Second, it allows clinicians to view a particular scale when they are reading reports of studies that use the measure. Many of the scales included in this book are reproduced in their entirety while the rest are summarized with references as to where the scale can be obtained.

This book is divided into several sections. The first section is an introduction on the use of assessment scales in clinical practice, providing a background and rationale for incorporating systematic assessment in the clinical care of patients with mood and anxiety disorders. Following is the main section containing the various scales separated into chapters focusing on depression and mania, anxiety, and depression and anxiety together, and special populations (child and adolescent, geriatric and medically ill groups). For these chapters we identified relevant instruments using a comprehensive search through the literature, focusing on scales that specifically relate to the measurement of severity and outcome rather than on diagnostic or screening tools. A few scales are included for historic reasons but otherwise we chose to include only those scales that we considered useful in current clinical practice.

We also include a chapter for related symptoms, side effects, psychosocial functioning and quality of life. This chapter includes several scales useful for measuring specific residual and associated symptoms of depression or anxiety and some of the side effects of medications. Additionally, in recognition of the importance of return to premorbid psychosocial functioning as an objective of treatment, we include scales that assess functional status and quality of life. In contrast to the earlier chapters, these are not meant to be a comprehensive selection of scales. Instead, we include a few selected scales for the most important residual symptoms such as sleep, pain and fatigue. These symptoms tend to be the ones most closely associated with non-adherence with treatment or to psychosocial impairment such as work disability. Similarly, the scales for side effects focus on those that are relevant but difficult to assess, such as sexual dysfunction or extrapyramidal symptoms.

Finally, we end with an index that lists all the scales in tabular form which summarizes important scale characteristics so that clinicians can choose an appropriate scale for a specific clinical indication or situation.

We thank our office staff, in particular Andrew Boylan, for the administrative work associated with the literature search and compilation of scales, and Abigail Griffin and Peter Stevenson for editorial guidance in producing this book.

Raymond W. Lam
Erin E. Michalak
Richard P. Swinson

Chapter 1

Why use assessment scales in clinical practice?

It has long been recognized in psychiatric research that measuring symptom severity across time is helpful in evaluating the course of treatment for psychiatric conditions. For example, all published clinical trials involve measuring outcome by means of scales focused on symptoms of interest. Rating symptoms is also an essential feature of newer psychological treatments such as cognitive-behavioural therapy. Yet, the use of assessment scales has not historically been a routine aspect of patient care for front-line mental health clinicians. In part, this may be due to the influence of psychodynamic psychotherapy, where the understanding of the patient was based primarily on understanding individual traits and where symptoms were only recognized as part of an underlying conflict or dynamic. It may also be because many clinicians (especially physicians, nurses, and social workers) are not trained in the use of assessment scales. Additionally, the nature of clinical practice with the pressure of high patient flow makes it difficult to incorporate yet more tasks into every patient encounter.

However, several recent developments have emphasized that using assessment scales should become a priority for clinicians. First, evidence-based medicine (EBM) has become the prevailing clinical framework for mental health. EBM promotes the use of evidence-based guidelines for clinical interventions and many of these guidelines offer treatment options based on scores from assessment scales. Second, there is much more emphasis on patient self-education and self-management, which includes self-monitoring of symptoms. Third, there is increasing recognition of the importance of residual or subsyndromal symptoms as predictors of poor outcome. These symptoms may not be detected unless an assessment scale is used. Finally, a cornerstone of EBM involves measuring the effectiveness of one's clinical practice. It is no longer sufficient to evaluate patient or practice outcomes by asking general questions about clinical status.

We can illustrate some of the clinical situations where assessment scales are helpful by comparing the practices of two prototypical clinicians, Dr Gestalt and Dr Scales. Dr Gestalt has always relied on his clinical acumen and a global opinion of how his patient is doing. Dr Scales, however, has incorporated the routine use of rating scales in her clinical practice. Both clinicians use clinical practice guidelines to guide their treatment decisions.

In the first clinical situation, they each see a patient with hand washing symptoms consistent with obsessive-compulsive disorder (OCD). Dr Gestalt determines the overall severity of the hand washing rituals and the germ obsessions, and initiates medication treatment with an SSRI while making a referral to a behavioural therapy clinic. Dr Gestalt is then puzzled when his patient does not return for follow-up and did not take the prescribed medication. Dr Scales, however, uses the Yale-Brown Obsessive Compulsive Scale during her assessment of the patient. By systematically covering the different types of OCD symptoms, she finds that the patient also has significant symptoms involving checking and counting rituals that interfere with taking the medication. Dr Scales is then able to use this information and enlist the help of a family member to administer the medication at home. In this situation, using an assessment scale led to a more thorough assessment and ensured that significant clinical symptoms are not missed.

In another clinical situation, each clinician assesses a patient with depression. They each make a clinical diagnosis of major depressive disorder, initiate treatment with an antidepressant medication, and book a follow-up appointment after 4 weeks. At the follow-up visit, Dr Gestalt asks his patient, 'How are you doing?' 'Terrible,' she replies, 'I don't feel any better than when I started the medication.' Checking his guidelines, Dr Gestalt decides to increase the dose of the antidepressant because of the lack of response at 4 weeks.

In contrast, Dr Scales uses the 17-item Hamilton Depression Rating Scale (HDRS) in her assessment. At baseline, her patient had an HDRS score of 25, putting her in the moderately to markedly depressed range. At the follow-up appointment, Dr Scales' patient says exactly the same thing, 'I don't feel any better than when I started the medication.' However, by using the HDRS to rate specific symptoms, Dr Scales finds out that her patient over the past week had slight improvement in sleep and appetite, slightly greater interest in her usual activities and was able to read more easily, resulting in an HDRS score of 19. These changes were not apparent to the patient because her mood had not yet improved. She still had negative cognitions associated with depression and globally felt no better. Despite the lack of subjective mood improvement, however, her HDRS score decreased from baseline by 25%. Checking her clinical guidelines, Dr Scales determines that this mild degree of improvement in symptoms merits a little more time on the same dose of medication. After another 4 weeks, the patient's HDRS score continued to improve and she began to notice that she was, indeed, feeling better. In this situation, using the HRDS changed the clinical decision and averted an unnecessary increase in the dose of medication.

Let's consider another clinical scenario with the same patient. Again, both Dr Gestalt and Dr Scales prescribe antidepressant medications for depression. A couple of months later, on a reassessment visit, Dr Gestalt asks his patient, 'How are you doing?' His patient replies, 'I'm doing very well and feeling much better'. Dr Gestalt gives himself a mental pat on his back and maintains the patient on the same dose of medication. He is then surprised when his patient returns two months later, saying that her symptoms are much worse, and it is clear that she has suffered a clinical relapse.

Meanwhile, Dr Scales has been using her HDRS in practice. After 8 weeks of treatment, her patient also says that she is feeling much better. However, on going through the HDRS, it is apparent that she still has some mild disturbances in sleep and energy, and that her concentration and memory have not yet returned to normal. Her HDRS score is still 10, clearly improved from her baseline score of 22 but not yet in full remission (commonly accepted as HDRS score of 7 or less). Recognizing that she still has residual symptoms of depression, Dr Scales continues to follow her closely. She increases the dose of the medication until a full response occurs and her HDRS scores fall into the normal range. She does well through the maintenance period and has no relapse of depression.

In this clinical vignette, keeping track of symptoms with an assessment scale has helped determine that residual symptoms are still present even though a substantial clinical response has occurred. Residual symptoms of depression are associated with poor outcomes, including increased risks of relapse, chronicity, suicide, and poor functioning. Hence, the therapeutic target for acute treatment of depression is now full symptom remission. A global assessment, however, often is not detailed or sensitive enough to detect residual symptoms. Dr Scales knows that certain residual symptoms, such as fatigue, pain, and daytime somnolence, are particularly associated with poor response or early relapse of depression. Using a validated assessment scale makes it much more likely that she will

be able to properly assess and monitor these important residual symptoms.

Obviously, a score on an assessment scale should not be the only factor considered when making these clinical decisions, just as a laboratory test cannot substitute for a clinical evaluation. A good clinician will appropriately ask the patient about specific symptoms of depression to determine the degree of clinical improvement. However, a rating scale can make this assessment more systematic and efficient.

Dr Gestalt often complains that he does not have enough time in a brief assessment visit to use a detailed rating scale. For this situation, brief interviewer-rated scales and/or self-rated scales can help to make a clinician's practice more efficient. For example, the 7-item version of the HDRS can provide a quick measure of clinical improvement in less than ten minutes. Alternatively, patients can complete a self-rated depression scale such as the Patient Health Questionnaire-9 (PHQ-9) at home, in the waiting room, or before a clinical encounter. The clinician can then quickly look over the results and focus in on the symptoms of most concern. Dr Scales finds that using assessment scales actually makes her more efficient and saves her time during a clinical visit.

Rating scales may also be beneficial to detect symptoms that are difficult to assess during a brief visit. Dr Scales recognizes that some of her patients feel more comfortable admitting certain symptoms, such as suicidal thoughts, in a questionnaire format rather than directly to her. She also uses assessment scales to monitor side effects to treatment, especially more sensitive ones such as sexual dysfunction. Many medication side effects can mimic the symptoms of anxiety or depression, hence she uses a side effects scale both before and during treatment. Other side effects, such as extrapyramidal symptoms associated with antipsychotic medications, are subtle and may be easily missed. A systematic approach that includes the use of rating scales is important for early detection and monitoring of these side effects that are critical factors in non-adherence.

Finally, evidence-based psychological treatments for depressive and anxiety disorders, such as cognitive-behavioural therapy (CBT), rely on rating scales as an integral part of the clinical assessment and follow-up. When Dr Gestalt refers a patient for CBT, he knows that a cornerstone of CBT is using a rating scale (e.g., the Beck Depression Inventory) to monitor treatment outcome. However, Dr Gestalt may not be aware of the increasing availability of chronic disease management (CDM) programs for primary care management of depressive and anxiety disorders. CDM programs focus on patient self-management strategies to develop an active therapeutic alliance with health care providers, including the use of patient-rated outcome scales. Dr Gestalt can reinforce and promote self-management by incorporating an assessment scale into his care plans so that his patients can self-monitor results of treatment.

Of course, there are important caveats and questions to consider in using assessment scales. What is the scale designed to measure? How effective is it at carrying out that task? What is the interval of assessment (today, past week, past month, etc.)? Is the scale clinician-administered, or can it be completed by the patient? Many scales require training for proper administration. Copyright issues dictate that some scales must be purchased for clinical use. Other scales are in the public domain and can be used freely. Users of self-rating scales must consider the unique characteristics of the patient – can they read the language, do they understand the questions, is there any cognitive impairment, are there psychiatric reasons why the patient might over- or under-endorse symptoms, etc. Users of interviewer-rated scales must consider issues such as inter-rater reliability and whether scoring conventions and rules are followed. Unstructured interviews are usually the least reliable among different raters, while structured or semi-structured interviews increase reliability by providing standardized questions for patients to answer.

Explicit and clear anchor points for each item also improve reliability of assessment scales.

In summary, the therapeutic objective for the treatment of anxiety and depression is full recovery, which includes the full remission of symptoms and a return to pre-morbid psychosocial functioning. Assessment scales are useful to assess clinical symptoms, monitor response to treatment and return of functioning, promote self-management strategies, detect residual symptoms, and ensure that side effects are not limiting treatment. Incorporating assessment scales into routine clinical practice means that treatment decisions can be made based on the best available information. For clinicians, the use of brief clinician-rated scales and/or patient-rated scales can improve the quality and efficiency of their clinical assessments. For patients, systematically tracking outcomes can provide valuable feedback on the effect of clinical interventions as an important component of self-management programmes and evidence-based psychotherapies. In this way, assessment scales can serve to enhance the therapeutic alliance and to promote adherence to both psychological and pharmacological treatment.

Chapter 2

Depression and mania

Mood disorders make up the most common psychiatric conditions in the population and account for a significant burden for individuals and on society. Depressive disorders include major depressive disorder (MDD), dysthymic disorder, and so-called 'minor depression'. Bipolar disorder consists of at least one manic or hypomanic episode in addition to depressive episodes.

Major depressive episode

The symptom criteria for a major depressive episode are similar in DSM-IV-TR and ICD-10 (Table 2.1). The symptoms of depression can be divided into cognitive/emotional (low mood, loss of interest or enjoyment, trouble concentrating, feelings of guilt or self-blame, thoughts of death and suicide) and vegetative (fatigue, psychomotor changes, disturbances of sleep and appetite/weight).

Dysthymic disorder refers to a low-grade, chronic form of depression. Fewer symptoms are required for the diagnosis compared to MDD but the symptoms must have been present for two years or longer. Cognitive symptoms (difficulty concentrating, feelings of guilt) are more common in dysthymia than are vegetative symptoms. Patients with dysthymia are also likely to experience periodic episodes of MDD. These 'double depressions' are often what leads patients to seek care. Dysthymia is seen more frequently in primary care settings than in specialty (psychiatry) clinics.

Although dysthymia and minor depression are often considered 'subsyndromal' depression, there is evidence that these conditions lead to significant morbidity and impairment of functioning, as well as being predictive of future episodes of MDD. Similarly, residual symptoms of depression, even when they do not meet criteria for MDD or dysthymia, are associated with poor outcomes such as risk of relapse into MDD, chronic courses of depression, poor psychosocial functioning, and suicide.

Subtypes of major depressive disorder

Major depressive disorder can also be divided into different 'subtypes', termed specifiers in DSM-IV-TR. These subtypes are classified according to the specific symptoms that are present during an episode (episode specifiers) or to the pattern of depressive episodes (course specifiers). The clinical importance of differentiating these subtypes is that treatment approach may vary according to subtype of depression (Table 2.2).

Melancholic specifier overlaps 'typical' depression with primary symptoms of non-reactive mood, in which the mood does not lift, even temporarily, when something good happens to the person, or loss of pleasure in all or almost all enjoyable activities. Melancholia also includes symptoms of insomnia, particularly terminal insomnia (with early morning wakening), diurnal variability in mood (with morning worsening), and marked appetite and weight loss.

In contrast, patients with atypical specifier present with a reactive mood state (where mood can improve transiently in response to something good that happens) and symptoms including leaden paralysis (a severe form of lethargy where arms and legs feel like lead), hyperphagia (overeating, often with carbohydrate craving and binge

---

Table 2.1 Summary of DSM-IV-TR symptom criteria for major depressive episode

- depressed mood, as indicated by either subjective report (e.g., feels sad or empty) or observation (e.g., appears tearful).
- markedly reduced interest or pleasure in all, or almost all, activities.
- significant weight loss when not dieting or weight gain (e.g., a change of more than 5% of body weight in a month), or decrease or increase in appetite.
- insomnia or hypersomnia (or increased need for sleep).
- psychomotor agitation or retardation (observable by others, not merely subjective feelings of restlessness or being slowed down).
- fatigue or loss of energy.
- feelings of worthlessness or excessive or inappropriate guilt (which may be delusional), not merely self-reproach or guilt about being sick.
- reduced ability to think or concentrate, or indecisiveness
- recurrent thoughts of death, recurrent suicidal ideation without a specific plan, or a suicide attempt or a specific plan for committing suicide.

Table 2.2 'Subtypes' of depression with clinical implications

Episode specifier	Key features	Clinical consideration
• Melancholic features	• Non-reactive mood state or anhedonia • Distinct quality of depressed mood, morning worsening of mood, early morning wakening, marked psychomotor changes, significant anorexia or weight loss, excessive or inappropriate guilt.	• Often more severe. • May be more likely to respond to biological interventions.
• Atypical features	• Reactive mood state. • Oversleeping, increased appetite and weight gain, leaden paralysis, interpersonal rejection sensitivity.	• Associated with early age of onset, chronic course and history of trauma/abuse. • MAOIs more effective than TCAs.
• Psychotic features	• Presence of hallucinations or delusions (especially delusions of guilt).	• Antidepressant + atypical antipsychotic agent. • Electroconvulsive therapy.
• Catatonic features	• Presence of catatonic signs and symptoms (elective mutism, rigidity, waxy flexibility, psychomotor excitation).	• Acute catatonia responds to injectible lorazepam or antipsychotic agents.

Course specifier	Key features	Clinical consideration
• Seasonal (winter) pattern	• Regular onset of depressive episodes during the fall/winter with summer remissions. • Atypical features such as oversleeping, overeating with carbohydrate craving, weight gain.	• Bright light therapy or antidepressant.
• Postpartum onset	• Onset of depressive episode within 4 weeks postpartum. • May be associated with psychotic features.	• Consider breastfeeding issues with pharmacotherapy.
• Rapid cycling	• 4 or more episodes of mania/hypomania and depression (or switches between states) in a year.	• Lithium less effective than anticonvulsants.

eating), hypersomnia (or increased need for sleep), and interpersonal rejection sensitivity (a personality trait in which people are extremely sensitive to real or perceived rejection, particularly romantic rejection). Atypical depression is actually quite common, affecting up to 40% of patients with MDD. It is also associated with early age of onset, chronic course, and history of trauma or abuse.

Other episode specifiers include psychotic depression with features such as hallucinations and/or delusional beliefs. Often these psychotic symptoms have self-critical content. Delusions of guilt are particularly common and may be missed unless specifically asked about. For example, these patients may believe that they are responsible for traffic accidents or natural disasters, or that they are being punished for their past actions. Finally, catatonic subtype is not commonly encountered in clinical practice, but this specifier includes features of catatonia (disturbances of psychomotor functioning) such as rigidity, elective mutism, waxy flexibility or psychomotor agitation/excitement.

People with depression worry and ruminate over problems and will usually have significant anxiety features. Anxiety disorders are frequently comorbid with depression, but even when syndromal disorders are not present, patients often have many symptoms of anxiety, including panic attacks, obsessions/compulsions, social anxiety, and generalized anxiety. A clinical picture of mixed anxiety and depression, where criteria are not met for either disorder, is particularly common in primary care practices. Although not considered a specific subtype of depression, some clinical practice guidelines have included evidence-based treatment recommendations for 'anxious depression' (Kennedy et al, 2001).

Course specifiers include seasonal pattern, otherwise known as seasonal affective disorder. These depressions only occur during a particular time of year. The usual pattern is winter depression, where patients have recurrent major depressive episodes in the fall and winter, with periods of normal mood in the spring and summer. Although the diagnosis is based on the pattern of episodes, patients with winter depression also commonly have atypical features, particularly the vegetative symptoms of fatigue, overeating and oversleeping.

Mania

Foremost in the differential diagnosis of depression is bipolar disorder, as indicated by a history of manic (type 1) or hypomanic (type 2) episodes. The symptoms of a manic episode include elevated mood or irritability, hyperactivity, grandiosity, rapid speech and thinking, distractibility, increased psychomotor activity, and decreased need for sleep (Table 2.3). Psychotic symptoms, including grandiose and religious delusions, paranoid ideation, ideas of reference or hallucinations, are often seen in more severe episodes.

Table 2.3 Summary of DSM-IV-TR symptom criteria for mania

- A distinct period of abnormally and persistently elevated, expansive, or irritable mood, lasting at least 1 week (or any duration if hospitalization is necessary).
- inflated self-esteem or grandiosity.
- decreased need for sleep (e.g., feels rested after only 3 hours of sleep).
- more talkative than usual or pressure to keep talking.
- flight of ideas or subjective experience that thoughts are racing.
- distractibility (i.e., attention too easily drawn to unimportant or irrelevant external stimuli).
- increase in goal-directed activity (either socially, at work or school, or sexually) or psychomotor agitation.
- excessive involvement in pleasurable activities that have a high potential for painful consequences (e.g., engaging in unrestrained buying sprees, sexual indiscretions, or foolish business investments).
- Note: Manic-like episodes that are clearly caused by somatic antidepressant treatment (e.g., medications, electroconvulsive therapy, light therapy) should not count toward a diagnosis of Bipolar I Disorder.

Manic episodes are defined as involving marked impairment in functioning and usually require hospitalization. Hypomania is a less severe form, defined with fewer symptoms to a less severe degree that results in less psychosocial impairment. Many patients with bipolar disorder initially present with depressive episodes. Treatment with an antidepressant can induce a manic or hypomanic episode, hence the importance of recognizing this condition.

Although the diagnosis of bipolar disorder is based on the presence of mania or hypomania, it is increasingly clear that depression is a greater clinical problem for patients with bipolar disorder. Over the course of the illness, patients with bipolar disorder spend much more time in syndromal and subsyndromal depressive episodes than manic or hypomanic episodes. The disability and psychosocial impairment associated with bipolar disorder is related much more to depression than mania. There is some evidence that depression in bipolar disorder is more likely to include atypical features, the so-called hypersomnic, anergic bipolar depression.

Increasing attention is also being paid to 'bipolar spectrum' disorders, characterized by subsyndromal symptoms of hypomania. These include brief episodes that do not meet the criteria for hypomania (e.g., 1 or 2 days of symptoms, or mood swings within a day), cyclothymia (in which there are frequent swings into mild depression or mild hypomania, with few periods of normal mood), and hypomanic symptoms that only occur during treatment with antidepressants. There is some evidence that these patients may not respond as well to antidepressants in the long term as these medications may induce rapid cycling. There is current controversy as to whether mood stabilizers are preferred treatments for bipolar spectrum conditions.

Bech–Rafaelsen Mania Scale (MAS)

Reference: **Bech P, Rafaelsen OJ, Kramp P, Bolwig TG. The mania rating scale: scale construction and inter-observer agreement. Neuropharmacology 1978; 17(6):430–1**

Rating Clinician-rated

Administration time 10 minutes

Main purpose To assess severity of symptoms of mania in patients with bipolar disorder

Population Adults and adolescents

Commentary

The MAS (also referred to in the literature as the BRMS, BRMAS or MRS) is an 11-item clinician-rated scale developed to assess symptoms of mania over the previous 3 days (or other specified time period) in patients with bipolar disorder. The MAS has been widely used as an outcome measure in treatment trials for bipolar disorder, particularly in Europe, and shows sound psychometric properties (see Bech, 2002, for review). For example, the scale demonstrates good inter-rater reliability, validity and responsiveness (it has been shown to be superior to the Clinical Global Impression Scale, see page 126, in terms of responsiveness to treatment, Bech et al., 2001). The MAS may be combined with Bech–Rafaelsen Melancholia Scale (see page 9) giving rise to the Bech–Rafaelsen Mania-Melancholia Scale (BRMMS).

Scoring

Items are scored on a 0 to 4 basis, yielding a total score range of 0–44, with higher scores indicating greater severity of mania. Scores in the range of 0–5 indicate no mania; 6–9 doubtful mania; 10–14 hypomania; 15–20 mild mania: 21–28 moderate mania; 29–44 severe (psychotic) mania.

Versions

The MAS has been translated into: Chinese, Danish, Dutch, English, Finnish, French, Greek, Italian, Norwegian, Polish, Portuguese, Russian, Spanish, Swedish and Turkish.

Additional references

Bech P, Baastrup PC, de Bleeker E, Ropert R. Dimensionality, responsiveness and standardization of the Bech–Rafaelsen Mania Scale in the ultra-short therapy with antipsychotics in patients with severe manic episodes. Acta Psychiatr Scand 2001; 104(1):25–30.

Bech P. The Bech–Rafaelsen Mania Scale in clinical trials of therapies for bipolar disorder: a 20-year review of its use as an outcome measure. CNS Drugs 2002; 16(1):47–63.

Bech P. The Bech–Rafaelsen Mania and Melancholia Scales in clinical trials: A 25-year review of their use as outcome measure in bipolar and unipolar patients In: Progress on Bipolar Disorder Research. Malcomb R. Brown (Editor) Nova Science Publishers, Inc., 2004.

Address for correspondence

Dr. Per Bech
WHO Collaborating Centre for Mental Health
Psychiatric Research Unit
Frederiksborg General Hospital
48, Dyrehavevej, DK-3400 Hillerød, Denmark
Telephone: 45 48 29 32 53
Email: pebe@fa.dk

The Bech–Rafaelsen Mania Scale (MAS)

No.	Symptom	Score
1	Elevated mood	0–4
2	Increased verbal activity	0–4
3	Increased social contact (intrusiveness)	0–4
4	Increased motor activity	0–4
5	Sleep disturbances	0–4
6	Social activities (distractibility)	0–4
7	Hostility, irritable mood	0–4
8	Increased sexual activity	0–4
9	Increased self-esteem	0–4
10	Flight of thoughts	0–4
11	Noise level	0–4
	Total score	0–44

Mania	MAS total score
Mild	15–20
Moderate	21–28
Severe	29–44

Reproduced from Bech P, Rafaelsen OJ, Kramp P, Bolwig TG. Neuropharmacology 1978; 17(6):430–1 by kind permission of Per Bech.

Bech–Rafaelsen Melancholia Rating Scale (MES)

Reference: **Bech P, Rafaelsen OJ. The use of rating scales exemplified by a comparison of the Hamilton and the Bech-Rafaelsen Melancholia Scale. Acta Psychiatr Scand Suppl 1980; 62(285):128–32**

Rating Clinician-rated

Administration time 10 minutes

Main purpose To assess severity of depressive symptoms

Population Adults and adolescents

Commentary

The MES (also referred to as the BRMS or BRMES) is an 11-item clinician-rated scale that represents an extensive modification of the Hamilton Rating Scale for Depression (see page 28). The scale assesses severity of depressive symptoms over the previous 3 days (or other specified time period). The instrument appears to show reasonable psychometric properties (moderate reliability, but good correlation with other depression rating scales such as Raskin Depression Rating Scale, see page 50). The uni-dimensionality of the MES has been confirmed in patients with major depression by different methodological approaches including Rasch analysis. Furthermore, the scale is able to discriminate major depression with melan-cholic features as opposed to depression without melan-cholia. The MES may be combined with Bech–Rafaelsen Mania Scale (see page 8) giving rise to the Bech–Rafaelsen Mania-Melancholia Scale (BRMMS).

Scoring

Items are scored on a 0 to 4 basis, yielding a total score range of 0–44, with higher scores indicating greater severity of depression. The scale developers suggest that scores in the range of 0–5 indicate no depression; 6–9, doubtful depression; 10–14, minor depression; 15–20, mild depression; 21–28, moderate depression; 29–44, severe (psychotic) depression.

Versions

The MES has been translated into: Chinese, Danish, Dutch, English, Finnish, French, Greek, Italian, Norwegian, Portuguese, Spanish and Swedish.

Additional references

Smolka M, Stieglitz RD. On the validity of the Bech–Rafaelsen Melancholia Scale (BRMS). J Affect Disord 1999; 54(1–2):119–28.

Bech P. The Bech–Rafaelsen Melancholia Scale (MES) in clinical trials of therapies in depressive disorders: a 20-year review of its use as outcome measure. Acta Psychiatr Scand 2002; 106(4):252–64.

Bent-Hansen J, Lunde M, Klysner R, Andersen M, Tanghøj P, Solstad K, Bech P. The validity of the depression rating scales in discriminating between citalopram and placebo in depression recurrence in the maintenance therapy of elderly unipolar patients with major depression. Pharmacopsychiatry 2003; 36(6):313–16

Bech P. The Bech–Rafaelsen Mania and Melancholia Scales in clinical trials: A 25-year review of their use as outcome measure in bipolar and unipolar patients. In: Progress on Bipolar Disorder Research. Malcomb R. Brown (Editor) Nova Science Publishers, Inc., 2004.

Address for correspondence

Dr. Per Bech
WHO Collaborating Centre for Mental Health
Psychiatric Research Unit
Frederiksborg General Hospital
48, Dyrehavevej, DK-3400 Hillerød, Denmark
Telephone: 45 48 29 32 53
Email: pebe@fa.dk

The Bech–Rafaelsen Melancholia Scale (MES)

No.	Symptom	Score
1	*Lowered mood	0–4
2	Decreased verbal activity	0–4
3	Decreased social contact	0–4
4	*Decreased motor activity	0–4
5	Sleep disturbances	0–4
6	*Decreased social activities	0–4
7	*Guilt feelings	0–4
8	*Tiredness	0–4
9	Suicidal thoughts	0–4
10	Poor concentration	0–4
11	*Anxiety	0–4
	Total score	0–44

*The six items of the melancholia subscale (MES-S)

Depression	MES total score
Mild	15–20
Moderate	21–28
Severe	29–44

Reproduced from Bech P, Rafaelsen OJ. Acta Psychiatr Scand Suppl 1980; 62(285):128–32 by kind permission of Per Bech.

Beck Depression Inventory – Second Edition (BDI-II)

Reference: **Beck AT, Steer RA, Brown GK. Manual for the BDI-II. 1996. San Antonio, TX, The Psychological Corporation**

Rating Self-report

Administration time 5–10 minutes

Main purpose To assess severity of depressive symptomatology

Population Adults and adolescents

Commentary

The gold standard of self-report depression rating scales, the BDI-II is a 21-item measure designed to assess DSM-IV defined symptoms of depression such as sadness, guilt, lost of interest, social withdrawal and suicidal ideation. Nineteen of the items are assessed on a 4-point scale according to increasing severity, with a further 2 items allowing the respondent to indicate increase or decrease in sleep or appetite (distinguishing it from the Beck Depression Inventory-IA, which did not assess atypical depressive symptoms). The instrument assesses the patient's mood and behaviour over the previous two weeks, and can be used either as a screening tool or to assess response to treatment. Given its brevity, ease of administration and relatively sound psychometric properties, the BDI-II remains one of the most popular self-report instruments for depression. It is worth noting that it has been criticized for discriminating poorly between depression and anxiety.

Scoring

Items are scored on a 0–3 scale, yielding a score range of 0–63 where higher scores indicate greater depression severity. According to Beck et al. (1996), scores in the range of 0–13 indicate minimal depression, 14–19 mild depression, 20–28 moderate depression, and 29–63 severe depression.

Versions

The scale has been translated into: Danish, Finnish, Flemish, French, Japanese, Portuguese and Spanish. A computer-administered version is available.

Additional references

Beck AT, Steer RA, Garbing MG. Psychometric properties of the Beck Depression Inventory: Twenty-five years of evaluation. Clin Psych Rev 1988; 8:77–100.

Richter P, Werner J, Heerlein A, Kraus A, Sauer H. On the validity of the Beck Depression Inventory. A review. Psychopathology 1998; 31(3):160–8.

Address for correspondence

Harcourt Assessment, Inc.
19500 Bulverde Road
San Antonio, TX 78259, USA
Telephone: 1-800-2111-8378
Website: www.HarcourtAssessment.com

Beck Hopelessness Scale (BHS)

Reference: **Beck AJ, Steer RA. Manual for the Beck Hopelessness Scale. 1988. San Antonio, TX, The Psychological Corporation**

Rating Self-report

Administration time 5–10 minutes

Main purpose To assess feelings of hopelessness about the future

Population Adults and adolescents

Commentary

The BHS is a 20-item self-report measure designed to assess peoples' feelings of hopelessness, specifically, their pessimism, loss of motivation and expectations about the future over the previous week. Responding either true or false to the items, patients can endorse a pessimistic statement or deny optimistic statements. Correlations have been shown between high BHS scores and depression, suicidal ideation, suicidal intent and eventual suicide. The BHS represents a rapid and useful probe for suicidal risk, although it is worth noting that hopelessness is not always correlated with suicidal behaviour, and the Beck Scale for Suicide Ideation (see page 12) may be a more direct method for assessing suicidal risk in some patients.

Scoring

Items are scored either 0 or 1, with a score range of 0–20, where higher scores indicate greater levels of hopelessness. Scores falling between 0–3 are considered within the normal range, 4–8 indicates mild hopelessness, 9–14 moderate, >14 severe.

Versions

The scale has been translated into: Chinese, Danish, Finnish and Portuguese. A computer-administered version is available.

Additional references

Beck AT, Brown G, Berchick RJ, Stewart BL, Steer RA. Relationship between hopelessness and ultimate suicide: a replication with psychiatric outpatients. Am J Psychiatry 1990; 147(2):190–5.

Beck AJ, Steer RA, Beck JS, Newman CF. Hopelessness, depression, suicidal ideation, and clinical diagnosis of depression. Suicide Life Threat Behav 1993; 23(2):139–45.

Address for correspondence

Harcourt Assessment, Inc.
19500 Bulverde Road
San Antonio, TX 78259, USA
Telephone: 1-800-2111-8378
Website: www.HarcourtAssessment.com

Beck Scale for Suicide Ideation (BSS)

Reference: **Beck AT, Steer RA. Beck Scale for Suicide Ideation: Manual. 1991. San Antonio, TX, The Psychological Corporation**

Rating Self-report

Administration time 5–10 minutes

Main purpose To assess suicide risk

Population Adults and adolescents

Commentary

The BSS is a 21-item self-report instrument developed to detect and measure intensity of suicidal ideation over the previous week. The questionnaire contains 5 initial screening items that reduce administration time in non-suicidal individuals. The remaining items address the patient's suicidal wishes, attitudes and plans, with 2 questions that assess number of previous suicide attempts and seriousness of intent to die in the most recent attempt. Although the BSS shows good reliability and internal consistency, the clinician-rated version of the scale (see below) has not been shown to predict ultimate suicide in patients who were longitudinally followed for a 10-year period (Beck et al., 1985). In other research, however, suicidal ideation has been shown to be related to likelihood of suicide attempt after discharge from hospital (Malone et al., 1995). The BSS provides a brief measure of suicide risk, to be used in conjunction with other clinical assessment tools.

Scoring

Items 1–19 are scored 0, 1 or 2 and summed, yielding a score range of 0–38. Higher scores indicate greater severity of suicidal ideation.

Versions

An earlier, clinician-rated version of the BSS (the Scale for Suicide Ideation or SSI) is available in two forms: the SSI-C (for current suicidal ideation) and the SSI-W (which rates worst suicidal ideation during the patient's lifetime). The BSS has been translated into Portuguese, and a computer-administered version is available.

Additional references

Beck AT, Steer RA, Kovacs M, Garrison B. Hopelessness and eventual suicide: a 10-year prospective study of patients hospitalized with suicidal ideation. Am J Psychiatry 1985; 142(5):559–63.

Malone KM, Haas GL, Sweeney JA, Mann JJ. Major depression and the risk of attempted suicide. J Affect Disord 1995; 34(3):173–85.

Beck AT, Brown GK, Steer RA. Psychometric characteristics of the Scale for Suicide Ideation with psychiatric outpatients. Behav Res Ther 1997; 35(11):1039–46.

Address for correspondence

Harcourt Assessment, Inc.
19500 Bulverde Road
San Antonio, TX 78259, USA
Telephone: 1-800-2111-8378
Website: www.HarcourtAssessment.com

Carroll Depression Scales–Revised (CDS-R)

Reference: **Carroll B. The Carroll Depression Scales: Technical Manual. 1998. Toronto, Canada, Multi-Health Systems Inc**

Rating Self-report

Administration time 20 minutes

Main purpose To assess severity of depressive symptoms

Population Adults

Commentary

The CDS-R is a 61-item self-report measure designed to assess severity of depressive symptomatology in concordance with the clinician-rated Hamilton Depression Rating Scale (HDRS) and DSM-IV. The scale allows the assessment of symptoms of MDD, dysthymia and melancholic and atypical symptoms. Items are structured in a yes/no format and patients are asked to think about how they have been feeling over the past few days. The CDS-R correlates well with other popular depression rating scales such as the Beck Depression Inventory (see page 10) and is appropriate for both assessing baseline depressive symptoms and monitoring change over time. A brief version (the 12-item Brief CDS) is also available for rapid screening.

Scoring

Items are scored either 0 or 1, yielding a score range of 0–61, where higher scores indicate higher levels of depression. Carroll et al. (1981) suggest a cut-off score of 10 when the CDS-R is used as a screening instrument.

Versions

The scale has been translated into French-Canadian.

Additional references

Carroll BJ, Feinberg M, Smouse PE, Rawson SG, Greden JF. The Carroll rating scale for depression. I. Development, reliability and validation. Br J Psychiatry 1981; 138:194–200.

Senra C. Evaluation and monitoring of symptom severity and change in depressed outpatients. J Clin Psychol 1996; 52(3):317–24.

Address for correspondence

Multi-Health Systems Inc.
P.O. Box 950
North Tonawanda, NY 14120–0950, USA
Telephone: 1-800-456-3003 in the US or 1-416-492-2627 international
Email: customerservice@mhs.com
Website: www.mhs.com

Centre for Epidemiological Studies Depression Scale (CES-D)

Reference: **Radloff LS. The CES-D Scale: A self-report depression scale for research in the general population. Appl Psychol Med 1977; 1:385–401**

Rating Self-report

Administration time 10 minutes

Main purpose To assess depressive symptomatology in the general population

Population Adults and adolescents

Commentary

Designed primarily for epidemiological research, the CES-D is a 20-item self-report instrument that assesses severity of depressive symptoms over the past week on a 4-point scale. Although the tool has been used extensively in research studies, it has seen less use in clinical settings. Research has indicated, however, that it is a psychometrically sound screening instrument that may be particularly useful in older adults.

Scoring

Items are scored either 0–3 or 3–0, with a range of 0–60, where higher scores indicate greater depressive symptomatology. A standard cut-off score of 16 is used to detect possible cases of depression, although Thomas et al. (2001) have reported that this cut-point has low positive predictive power.

Versions

The scale has been translated into: Afrikaans, Arabic, Cambodian, Canadian French, Chinese for Hong Kong, Danish, Dutch, Dutch for Belgium, English for UK, French, French for Belgium, German, Greek, Italian, Japanese, Portuguese, Spanish and Swedish.

Additional references

Lyness JM, Noel TK, Cox C, King DA, Conwell Y, Caine ED. Screening for depression in elderly primary care patients. A comparison of the Center for Epidemiologic Studies-Depression Scale and the Geriatric Depression Scale. Arch Intern Med 1997; 157(4):449–54.

Thomas JL, Jones GN, Scarinci IC, Mehan DJ, Brantley PJ. The utility of the CES-D as a depression screening measure among low-income women attending primary care clinics. The Center for Epidemiologic Studies-Depression. Int J Psychiatry Med 2001; 31(1):25–40.

Address for correspondence

Epidemiology and Psychopathology Research Branch
Room 10C-05
National Institute of Mental Health
5600 Fishers Lane
Rockville, MD 20857, USA
Telephone: 1-301-443-3648/3774
Email: hlejnar@mail.nih.gov

Center for Epidemiological Studies Depression Scale (CES-D)

Circle the number for each statement which best describes how often you felt or behaved this way – DURING THE PAST WEEK

	Rarely or none of the time (less than 1 day)	Some or a little of the time (1–2 days)	Occasionally or a moderate amount of time (3–4 days)	Most or all of the time (5–7 days)
DURING THE PAST WEEK:				
1. I was bothered by things that usually don't bother me	0	1	2	3
2. I did not feel like eating; my appetite was poor	0	1	2	3
3. I felt that I could not shake off the blues even with help from my family or friends	0	1	2	3
4. I felt that I was just as good as other people	0	1	2	3
5. I had trouble keeping my mind on what I was doing	0	1	2	3
6. I felt depressed	0	1	2	3
7. I felt that everything I did was an effort	0	1	2	3
8. I felt hopeful about the future	0	1	2	3
9. I thought my life had been a failure	0	1	2	3
10. I felt fearful	0	1	2	3
11. My sleep was restless	0	1	2	3
12. I was happy	0	1	2	3
13. I talked less than usual	0	1	2	3
14. I felt lonely	0	1	2	3
15. People were unfriendly	0	1	2	3
16. I enjoyed life	0	1	2	3
18. I felt sad	0	1	2	3
19. I felt that people disliked me	0	1	2	3
20. I could not get 'going'	0	1	2	3

Reproduced from Radloff LS. Appl Psychol Med 1977; 1:385–401

Clinician-Administered Rating Scale for Mania (CARS-M)

Reference: Altman EG, Hedeker DR, Janicak PG, Peterson JL, Davis JM. The Clinician-Administered Rating Scale for Mania (CARS-M): development, reliability, and validity. Biol Psychiatry 1994; 36(2):124–34

Rating Clinician-rated

Administration time 15–30 minutes

Main purpose To assess severity of manic and psychotic symptoms

Population Adults

Commentary

The CARS-M is a 15-item clinician-rated scale designed to assess severity of both manic and psychotic symptoms over the previous week. The instrument yields 2 sub-scales: a mania scale and a separate scale for psychotic symptoms and disorganization. The instrument correlates well with the Young Mania Rating Scale (see page 57) and shows good reliability. It is worth noting that the CARS-M does not assess depressive symptoms, and that it may be necessary to concurrently administer a depression rating scale in patients with bipolar disorder.

Scoring

Items are scored on a 0–5 scale, with the exception of the insight item, which is rated on a 0–4 scale. Score range for the mania sub-scale is 0–50 and range for the psychosis sub-scale is 0–24, although the 2 scales can be combined to provide a total score for mania with psychotic features (range 0–74). The instrument provides clear anchor points and prompt questions. The following severity guidelines are provided for the mania sub-scale: 0–7 (no or questionable mania); 8–15 (mild mania); 16–25 (moderate mania); ≥26 (severe symptomatology).

Versions

The instrument has been translated into Spanish.

Additional reference

Poolsup N, Li Wan Po A, Oyebode F. Measuring mania and critical appraisal of rating scales. J Clin Pharm Ther 1999; 24(6):433–43.

Address for correspondence

Dr. Edward Altman
Psychiatric Institute
1601 West Taylor Street
Chicago, IL 60612, USA
Telephone: 1-312-355-1659
Email: Ealtman@psych.uic.edu

Clinician-Administered Rating Scale for Mania (CARS-M)

Patient _____ Date _____ Rater(s) _____

Mania subscale (items 1–10) _____ Psychosis subscale (items 11–15) _____ Total score _____

Note: In completing this scale, information may be obtained, not only from the patient interview, but also from reliable collateral sources, including: family, nursing staff, hospital records, etc. In general, the time period for assessing symptoms should be the last seven days, but may be longer if required.

1. **Elevated/Euphoric Mood** (Inappropriate optimism about the present or future which lasted at least several hours and was out of proportion to the circumstances.)
   - Have there been times in the past week/month when you felt unusually good, cheerful, or happy?
   - Did you feel as if everything would turn out just the way you wanted?
   - Is this different from your normal mood? How long did it last?
   0 Absent
   1 Slight, e.g., good spirits, more cheerful than others, of questionable clinical significance.
   2 Mild, but definitely elevated or expansive mood, overly optimistic and somewhat out of proportion to one's circumstances.
   3 Moderate, mood and outlook clearly out of proportion to circumstances.
   4 Severe, clear quality of euphoric mood.
   5 Extreme, clearly exhausted, extreme feelings of well being, inappropriate laughter and/or singing.

2. **Irritability/Aggressiveness** (Has recently demonstrated, inside or outside of the interview, **overt** expression of anger, irritability, or annoyance. Do not include mere subjective feelings of anger/annoyance, unless expressed overtly.)
   - How have you been getting along with people in general?
   - Have you been feeling irritable or angry? How much of the time?
   - Have you been involved in any arguments or fights? How often?
   0 Absent
   1 Slight, occasional annoyance, questionable clinical significance.
   2 Mild, somewhat argumentative, quick to express annoyance with patients, staff or inteviewer, occasionally irritable during interview.
   3 Moderate, often swears, loses temper, threatening, excessive irritation around certain topics, room seclusion may be required, frequently irritable during interview.
   4 Severe, occasionally assaultive, may throw objects, damage property, limit setting necessary, excessive and inappropriate irritation, restraints may be required, interview had to be stopped due to excessive irritability.
   5 Extreme, episodes of violence against persons or objects, physical restraint required.

3. **Hypermotor Activity** (Has recently demonstrated, inside or outside of the interview, visible manifestations of generalized motor hyperactivity. Do not include mere subjective feelings of restlessness – *not medication related.*)
   - Have there been times when you were unable to sit still or times when you had to be moving or pacing back and forth?
   0 Absent
   1 Slight increase, of doubtful clinical significance.
   2 Mild, occasional pacing, unable to sit quietly in chair.
   3 Moderate, frequent pacing on unit, unable to remain seated.
   4 Marked, almost constant moving or pacing about.
   5 Extreme, continuous signs of hyperactivity such that the patient must be restrained to avoid exhaustion.

4. **Pressured Speech** (Accelerated, pressured, or increased amount and rate of speech, inside or outside of the interview.)
   0 Absent
   1 Slight increase, of doubtful clinical significance.
   2 Mild, noticeably more verbose than normal, but conversation is not strained.
   3 Moderate, so verbose that conversation is strained; some difficulty interrupting patient's speech.
   4 Marked, patient's conversation is so rapid that conversation is difficult to maintain, markedly difficult to interrupt speech.
   5 Extreme, speech is so rapid or continuous that patient cannot be interrupted.

5. **Flight of Ideas/Racing Thoughts** (Accelerated speech with abrupt changes from topic to topic, usually based on understandable associations, distracting stimuli, or play on words. When severe, the associations may be so difficult to understand that looseness of association or incoherence may also be present. Racing thoughts refer to the patient's subjective report of having thoughts racing through his mind.)
   - Have you been bothered by having too many thoughts at one time?
   - Have you had thoughts racing through your mind? How often? Does it hinder your functioning?
   0 Absent
   1 Slight, occasional instances of doubtful clinical significance.
   2 Mild, occasional instances of abrupt change in the topic with little impairment in understandability or patient reports occasional racing thoughts.
   3 Moderate, frequent instances with some impairment in understandability or patient reports frequent racing thoughts which are disruptive or distressing to the patient.
   4 Severe, very frequent instances with definite impairment.
   5 Extreme, most of speech consists of rapid changes in topic which are difficult to follow.

6. **Distractibility** (Attention is too easily drawn to unimportant or irrelevant *external* stimuli; i.e., noise in adjoining room, books on a shelf, interviewer's clothing, etc. **Exclude** distractibility due to intrusions of visual and/or auditory hallucinations or delusions. Rate on the basis of **observation only**.)
   0 Absent
   1 Slight, of doubtful clinical significance.
   2 Mild, present but does not interfere with task or conversation.
   3 Moderate, some interference with conversation or task.
   4 Severe, frequent interference with conversation or task.
   5 Extreme, unable to focus patient's attention on task or conversation.

7. **Grandiosity** (Increased self-esteem and unrealistic or inappropriate appraisal of one's worth, value, power, knowledge or abilities.)
   - Have you felt more self-confident than usual?
   - Have you felt that you were a particularly important person or that you had special powers, knowledge or abilities that were out of the ordinary?
   - Is there a special mission or purpose to your life?
   - Do you have a special relationship with God?

0 Absent

1 Slightly increased self-esteem or confidence, but of questionable clinical significance.

2 Mild, definitely inflated self-esteem or exaggeration of abilities somewhat out of proportion to circumstances.

3 Moderate, inflated self-esteem clearly out of proportion to circumstances, borderline delusional intensity.

4 Severe, clear grandiose delusion(s).

5 Extreme, preoccupied with and/or acts on the basis of grandiose delusion(s).

8. **Decreased Need For Sleep** (Less need for sleep than usual to feel rested. Do **not** rate difficulty with initial, middle or late insomnia.)

   - How much sleep do you ordinarily need?
   - Have you needed less sleep than usual to feel rested?
   - How much less sleep do/did you need?

0 Absent

1 Up to 1 hour less sleep than usual.

2 Up to 2 hours less sleep than usual.

3 Up to 3 hours less sleep than usual.

4 Up to 4 hours less sleep than usual.

5 4 or more hours less sleep than usual.

9. **Excessive Energy** (Unusually energetic or more active than usual without expected fatigue, lasting at least several days, including increased sexual interest or energy.)

   - Have you had more energy than usual? Has your interest in sex increased?
   - Have you been more active (either socially or sexually) than usual, or had the feeling that you could go all day without feeling tired?

0 Absent

1 Slightly more energy or increased sexual interest, of questionable significance.

2 Definite increase in activity level or less fatigued than usual, does not hinder functioning.

3 Clearly more active than usual sexually or physically, with little or no fatigue, occasional interference with functioning.

4 Much more active sexually or physically than usual with little fatigue and clear interference with normal functioning.

5 Extreme, active all day long with little or no fatigue or need for sleep.

10. **Poor Judgement** (Excessive involvement in activities without recognizing the high potential for painful consequences; intrusiveness, inappropriate calling of attention to oneself.)

    - When you were feeling high/irritable, did you do things that caused trouble for you or your family?
    - Did you spend money foolishly?
    - Did you take on responsibilities for which you were unqualified?

0 Absent

1 Slight, but of questionable clinical significance (i.e. increased phone calling, occasional intrusiveness.)

2 Mild, but definite examples (i.e. somewhat intrusive, sexually provocative, inappropriate singing.)

3 Moderate, assumes tasks or responsibilities without proper training, financial indiscretions, buying sprees within financial limits, frequent intrusiveness.

4 Severe, sexual promiscuity, hypersexuality, extremely intrusive behavior, places self in significant economic difficulty.

5 Extreme, continuous intrusive behavior requiring limited setting, excessive phone calling at all hours, antisocial behavior, excessive involvement in activities without regard to consequences.

11. **Disordered Thinking** (Impaired understandability of patient's thoughts as manifested by his/her speech. This may be due to any one or a combination of the following; incoherence, looseness of association(s), neologisms, illogical thinking. Do **not** rate simple flight of ideas unless severe.)

0 Absent

1 Occasional instances which are of doubtful clinical significance.

2 A few definite instances, but little or no impairment in understandability.

3 Frequent instances and may have some impairment in understandability.

4 Severe, very frequent instances with marked impairment in understandability.

5 Extreme, most or all of speech is distorted, making it impossible to understand what the patient is talking about.

12. **Delusions** (Fixed false beliefs, ranging from delusional ideas to full delusions – **including grandiosity**)

    Specify type(s): _____.

    - Have you felt that anyone was trying to harm you or hurt you for no reason? Can you give an example?
    - Have you felt as if you were being controlled by an external force or power? (Example?)
    - Have you felt as if people on the radio or TV were talking to you, about you, or communicating to you in some special way? (Example.)
    - Have you had any (other) strange or unusual beliefs or ideas? (Example.)
    - Have these beliefs interfered with your functioning in any way? (Example.)

0 Absent

1 Suspected or likely.

2 Definitely present but not fully convicted, including referential or persecutory ideas without full conviction.

3 Definitely present with full conviction but little if any influence on behavior.

4 Delusion has a significant effect upon patient's thoughts, feelings, or behavior (i.e., preoccupied with belief that others are trying to harm him/her.)

5 Actions based on delusion have major impact on patient or others (i.e., stops eating due to belief that food is poisoned, strikes others due to beliefs that others are trying to harm him/her.)

13. **Hallucinations** (A sensory perception without external stimulation of the relevant sensory organ.)

    Specify type(s): _____.

    - Have you heard sounds or voices of people talking when there was no one around? (Example.)
    - Have you seen any visions or smelled odors that others don't seem to notice? (Example.)
    - Have you had any (other) strange or unusual perceptions? (Example.)
    - Have these experiences interfered with your functioning in any way? (Example.)

0 Absent

1 Suspected or likely.

2 Present, but subject is generally aware that it may be his/her imagination and can ignore it.

3 Definitely present with full conviction but little if any influence on behavior.

4 Hallucinations have significant effect on patient's thoughts, feelings, or actions (e.g., locks doors to avoid imaginary pursuers.)

5 Actions based on hallucinations have major impact on patient or others (e.g., patient converses with voices so much that it interferes with normal functioning.)

14. Orientation (Impairment in recent or remote memory, or disorientation to person, place or time.)
- Have you recently had trouble remembering who you were, the dates or current events?
- Do you know the day of the week, the month, the year, and the name of this place?

0 Absent

1 Slight impairment but of doubtful clinical significance (i.e., misses date by one day.)

2 Mild, but definite impairment (i.e., unsure about orientation to place or time, or some impairment in a few aspects of recent or remote memory.)

3 Moderate (i.e., confused about where he is or cannot remember many important events in his life.)

4 Severe (disoriented or gross impairment in memory.)

5 Extreme (i.e., thoroughly disoriented to time, place, person and/or is unable to recall numerous important events in his/her life.)

15. Insight (The extent to which patient demonstrates an awareness or understanding of their emotional illness, aberrant behavior and/or a corresponding need for psychiatric/psychological treatment.)
- Do you feel that you currently suffer from emotional or psychological problems of any kind?
- How would you explain your behavior or symptoms?
- Do you currently believe that you may need psychiatric treatment?

0 Insight is present (i.e., patient admits illness, behavior change and need for treatment.)

1 Partial insight is present (i.e., patient feels he/she may possibly be ill or needs treatment, but is unsure.)

2 Patient admits behavior change, illness or need for treatment but attributes it to non-delusional or plausable external factors (i.e., marital conflict, job difficulties, stress.)

3 Patient admits behavior change, illness or need for treatment but gives delusional explanations (i.e., being controlled by external forces, dying of cancer, etc.)

4 Complete lack of insight. Patient denies behavior change, illness or need for treatment.

Reprinted from Altman EG, Hedeker DR, Janicak PG, Peterson JL, Davis JM. Biol Psychiatry 1994; 36(2):124–34. © 1994, with permission from Society of Biological Psychiatry.

Cornell Dysthymia Rating Scale (CDRS)

Reference: **Mason BJ, Kocsis JH, Leon AC, Thompson S, Frances AJ, Morgan RO, Parides MK. Measurement of severity and treatment response in dysthymia. Psychiatr Ann 1993; 23(11):625–31**

Rating Clinician-rated

Administration time 20 minutes

Main purpose To assess severity of symptoms of dysthymia

Population Adults

Commentary

The CDRS is a 20-item clinician-rated scale developed specifically to assess severity of symptoms of dysthymia (chronic, mild depression). Raters are required to assess both frequency and severity of symptoms over the previous week. The CDRS has been shown to be sensitive to change in response to treatment, and provides a useful tool to monitor symptoms of dysthymia.

Scoring

Items are scored on a 0–4 basis, with a total score range of 0–80, where higher scores indicate greater severity of symptoms.

Versions

A self-report version is available.

Additional references

Cohen J. Assessment and treatment of dysthymia: The development of the Cornell Dysthymia Rating Scale. Eur Psychiatry 1997; 12(4):190–3.

Hellerstein DJ, Batchelder ST, Lee A, Borisovskaya M. Rating dysthymia: an assessment of the construct and content validity of the Cornell Dysthymia Rating Scale. J Affect Disord 2002; 71(1–3):85–96.

Address for correspondence

Dr. Barbara J. Mason
Alcohol Disorders Research Clinic
Department of Psychiatry & Behavioral Sciences
University of Miami/Jackson Memorial Medical Center
1400 N.W. 10th Avenue, Suite 307
Miami, FL 33136, USA
Telephone: 1-305-243-4644
Email: bjmason246@aol.com

Cornell Dysthymia Rating Scale (CDRS)

Instruction: Rate each item for the previous week

1. Depressed mood
Subjective feelings of depression based on verbal complaints of feeling depressed, sad, blue, gloomy, down in the dumps, empty, 'don't care'. Do not include such ideational aspects as discouragement, pessimism, and worthlessness or suicide attempts (all of which are to be rated separately).
- ☐ 0 – Not at all
- ☐ 1 – Slight, e.g. only occasionally feels 'sad' or 'down'
- ☐ 2 – Mild, e.g. often feels somewhat 'depressed', 'blue', or 'down-hearted'
- ☐ 3 – Moderate, e.g. most of the time feels depressed
- ☐ 4 – Severe, e.g. most of the time feels 'very depressed' or 'miserable'

2. Lack of interest or pleasure
Pervasive lack of interest in work, family, friends, sex, hobbies, and other leisure time activities. Severity is determined by the number of important activities in which the subject has less interest or pleasure compared to nonpatients.
- ☐ 0 – All activities as interesting or pleasurable
- ☐ 1 – 1 or 2 activities less interesting or pleasurable
- ☐ 2 – Several activities less interesting or pleasurable
- ☐ 3 – Most activities less interesting or pleasurable with one or two exceptions
- ☐ 4 – Total absence of pleasure in almost all activities

3. Pessimism
Discouragement, pessimism and hopelessness
- ☐ 0 – Not at all discouraged about the future
- ☐ 1 – Slight, e.g. occasional feelings of mild disappointment about the future
- ☐ 2 – Mild, e.g. often somewhat discouraged but can usually be talked into feeling hopeful
- ☐ 3 – Moderate, e.g. often feels quite pessimistic about the future and can only sometimes be talked into being hopeful
- ☐ 4 – Severe, e.g. pervasive feelings of intense pessimism or hopelessness

4. Suicidal tendencies
Suicidal tendencies, including preoccupation with thoughts of death or dying. Do not include mere fears of dying.
- ☐ 0 – Not at all
- ☐ 1 – Slight, e.g. occasionally feels life is not worth living
- ☐ 2 – Mild, e.g. frequent thoughts that s/he would be better off dead or occasional thoughts of wishing s/he were dead
- ☐ 3 – Moderate, e.g. often thinks of suicide, has thought of specific method, or made an impulsive attempt not requiring medical attention
- ☐ 4 – Severe, e.g. has made a planned attempt requiring medical intervention

5. Low self-esteem
Negative evaluation of self, including feelings of inadequacy, failure, worthlessness
- ☐ 0 – Not at all
- ☐ 1 – Slight, e.g. occasional feelings of inadequacy
- ☐ 2 – Mild, e.g. often feels somewhat inadequate
- ☐ 3 – Moderate, e.g. often feels like a failure
- ☐ 4 – Severe, e.g. constant, pervasive feelings of worthlessness

6. Guilt
Feelings of self-reproach or excessive, inappropriate guilt for things done or not done
- ☐ 0 – Not at all
- ☐ 1 – Slight, e.g. occasional feelings of mild self-blame
- ☐ 2 – Mild, e.g. often somewhat guilty about past actions, the significance of which s/he exaggerates, such as consequences of his/her illness
- ☐ 3 – Moderate, e.g. often feels quite guilty about past actions or feelings of guilt which s/he can't explain
- ☐ 4 – Severe, e.g. pervasive feelings of intense guilt or generalizes feelings of self-blame to many situations

7. Helplessness
Feelings of passivity, lack of control, needing someone's assistance to get mobilized
- ☐ 0 – Not at all
- ☐ 1 – Slight and of doubtful clinical significance
- ☐ 2 – Mild, e.g. of clinical significance, but only occasional and never very intense, effort to take initiative, but does so
- ☐ 3 – Moderate, e.g. often aware of feeling quite helpless or occasionally feeling very helpless; missed opportunities by not taking initiative; needs a lot of coaxing or reassurance
- ☐ 4 – Marked, e.g. most of the time feeling quite helpless or often feeling very helpless

8. Social withdrawal
Lack of social contact with persons out of the home
- ☐ 0 – Not at all
- ☐ 1 – Possibly less sociable than the norm
- ☐ 2 – At times definitely avoids socializing
- ☐ 3 – Often avoids friends and social interactions
- ☐ 4 – Almost all the time avoids interpersonal contacts

9. Indecisiveness
Difficulty making decisions
- ☐ 0 – Not at all
- ☐ 1 – Slight, e.g. occasional difficulty making decisions
- ☐ 2 – Mild, e.g. often has difficulty making decisions
- ☐ 3 – Moderate, e.g. frequently ruminates excessively and feels unsure when decision making
- ☐ 4 – Severe, e.g. usually unable to make even simply decisions in most situations

10 Low attention and concentration
Distractible, unfocused, confused thinking, impaired short-term memory
- ☐ 0 – Not at all
- ☐ 1 – Occasional mild distractibility
- ☐ 2 – At times definite difficulty concentrating
- ☐ 3 – Often has difficulty concentrating
- ☐ 4 – Almost all the time has significant difficulty paying attention and concentrating, e.g. cannot retain what is read

11. Psychic anxiety
Subjective feelings of anxiety, fearfulness, or apprehension, excluding anxiety attacks, whether or not accompanied by somatic anxiety, and whether focused on specific concerns or not
- ☐ 0 – Not at all
- ☐ 1 – Slight, e.g. occasionally feels somewhat anxious
- ☐ 2 – At times definitely anxious
- ☐ 3 – Moderate, e.g. most of the time feels anxious
- ☐ 4 – Severe, e.g. most of the time feels very anxious

12. **Somatic anxiety**
    Has been bothered by 1 or more physiological concomitants of anxiety other than during a panic attack. They include symptoms associated with panic attacks, as well as headaches, stomach cramps, diarrhea, or muscle tension. This item should be scored whether or not the subject has had panic attacks.
    - ☐ 0 – Not at all or only during anxiety attacks
    - ☐ 1 – Slight, e.g. occasionally palms sweating excessively
    - ☐ 2 – Mild, e.g. often has 1 or more physical symptoms to a mild degree
    - ☐ 3 – Moderate, e.g. often has several symptoms or symptoms to a considerable degree
    - ☐ 4 – Severe, e.g. very frequently is bothered by 2 or more symptoms

13. **Worry**
    Worrying, brooding, painful preoccupation and inability to get mind off unpleasant thoughts (may or may not be accompanied by depressive mood)
    - ☐ 0 – Not at all
    - ☐ 1 – Slight, e.g. occasionally worries about some realistic problem
    - ☐ 2 – Mild, e.g. often worries excessively about a realistic problem or occasionally about some trivial problem
    - ☐ 3 – Moderate, e.g. very often worries excessively about a realistic problem and often worries about some trivial problem
    - ☐ 4 – Severe, e.g. most of the time is spent in worrying or brooding

14. **Irritability or excessive anger**
    Feelings of anger, resentment, or annoyance (directed externally) whether expressed overly or not. Rate only the intensity and duration of the subjective mood.
    - ☐ 0 – Not at all
    - ☐ 1 – Slight, e.g. occasionally feels somewhat anxious
    - ☐ 2 – At times definitely feels anxious
    - ☐ 3 – Moderate, e.g. most of the time feels anxious
    - ☐ 4 – Severe, e.g. most of the time feels very anxious

15. **Somatic general**
    Physical symptoms such as heaviness in limbs, back, or head, backaches, muscle aches
    - ☐ 0 – Not at all
    - ☐ 1 – Slight, e.g. occasional backache
    - ☐ 2 – Mild, e.g. often has 1 or more physical symptoms to a mild degree
    - ☐ 3 – Moderate, e.g. often has 1 or more symptoms to a considerable degree
    - ☐ 4 – Severe, e.g. very frequently is bothered by 2 or more symptoms which interfere with function

16. **Low productivity**
    Decreased effectiveness or productivity at school, work, or home, as compared with nonpatients.
    - ☐ 0 – Not at all
    - ☐ 1 – Occasional decrease in functioning in 1 or 2 areas
    - ☐ 2 – Frequent decrease in functioning in 1 or 2 areas
    - ☐ 3 – Frequent decrease in functioning in several areas
    - ☐ 4 – Decrease in functioning in almost all areas a great deal of the time

17. **Low energy**
    Subjective feeling of lack of energy or fatigue. (Do not confuse with lack of interest.)
    - ☐ 0 – Not at all
    - ☐ 1 – Probably less energy than normal
    - ☐ 2 – At times definitely more tired or less energy than normal
    - ☐ 3 – Often feels tired or without energy
    - ☐ 4 – Almost all the time feels very tired or without energy or spends a great deal of time resting

18. **Low sexual interest, activity**
    - ☐ 0 – Not at all
    - ☐ 1 – Possibly less than normal
    - ☐ 2 – At times definitely low
    - ☐ 3 – Often low
    - ☐ 4 – Almost all the time

19. **Insomnia**
    Sleep disturbance, including difficulty in getting to sleep, staying asleep or sleeping too much. Take into account the estimated number of hours slept and subjective sense of adequacy of time spent sleeping. If subject is using medication, ask what he thinks it would be like without medication.
    Choose either A or B
    A Difficulty getting to sleep or staying asleep
    - ☐ 0 – Not at all
    - ☐ 1 – Slight, e.g. occasional difficulty
    - ☐ 2 – Mild, e.g. often has some significant difficulty
    - ☐ 3 – Moderate, e.g. usually has considerable difficulty
    - ☐ 4 – Severe, e.g. almost always has great difficulty
    B Sleeps too much
    - ☐ 0 – Not at all
    - ☐ 1 – Slight, e.g. occasional difficulty
    - ☐ 2 – Mild, e.g. often has some significant difficulty
    - ☐ 3 – Moderate, e.g. usually has considerable difficulty
    - ☐ 4 – Severe, e.g. almost always has great difficulty

20. **Diurnal mood variations**
    Extent to which, for at least 1 week, there is a constant fluctuation of depressed mood and other symptomatology coinciding with the first or second half of the day. Generally, if the mood is worse in one part of the day it will be better in the other. However, for occasional subjects who are better in the afternoon and worse in the morning and evening, choose the one time that represents the greatest severity of symptoms.
    Choose either A or B
    A Worse in morning
    - ☐ 0 – Not worse in morning or variable
    - ☐ 1 – Minimally or questionably worse
    - ☐ 2 – Mildly worse
    - ☐ 3 – Moderately worse
    - ☐ 4 – Considerably worse
    B Worse in evening
    - ☐ 0 – Not worse in evening or variable
    - ☐ 1 – Minimally or questionably worse
    - ☐ 2 – Mildly worse
    - ☐ 3 – Moderately worse
    - ☐ 4 – Considerably worse

Rater's name _____

Cornell Dysthymia Score _____

Diagnostic Inventory for Depression (DID)

Reference: **Zimmerman M, Sheeran T, Young D. The Diagnostic Inventory for Depression: A self-report scale to diagnose DSM-IV major depressive disorder. J Clin Psychol 2004; 60(1):87–110**

Rating Self-report

Administration time 15–20 minutes

Main purpose To diagnose depression according to DSM-IV criteria, and to assess psychosocial impairment and quality of life

Population Adults

Commentary

The recently developed DID is a 38-item self-report scale designed to assess DSM-IV defined symptoms of MDD, psychosocial impairment due to depression, and quality of life. Nineteen of the scale's questions assess severity of a comprehensive range of depressive symptoms over the past week, with a further 3 items assessing frequency of depressed mood, loss of interest in usual activities, or loss of pleasure in usual activities over the previous 2 weeks. The 6-item psychosocial functioning subscale evaluates the degree of difficulty depressive symptoms have caused in usual daily responsibilities, interpersonal relationships, participation in leisure activities, and overall functioning. The quality of life subscale assesses satisfaction with corresponding domains, in addition to global satisfaction with mental and physical health. The DID is unusual in that it concomitantly assesses persistence, duration and severity of depressive symptoms. An initial evaluation of its psychometric properties in a large sample of psychiatric outpatients has shown promising results, although more information is needed about the scale's responsiveness to change.

Scoring

All items except the 'loss of interest or pleasure in usual activities' questions are scored on a 0–4 scale, where a score of 0 = no disturbance, 1 = sub-clinical severity, and ≥ 2 indicates that the symptom is present. For the loss of interest or pleasure items, a score ≥ 3 indicates that the symptom is present. The DID uses an algorithmic approach (described in detail in the primary reference) to diagnosis of MDD that mirrors the DSM-IV diagnostic procedure.

Versions

No other versions are currently available.

Additional reference

Sheeran T, Zimmerman M. Case identification of depression with self-report questionnaires. Psychiatry Res 2002; 109(1):51–9.

Address for correspondence

Dr. Mark Zimmerman
Bayside Medical Building
235 Plain Street
Providence, RI 02905, USA
Telephone 1-401-277-0724
Email: Mzimmerman@lifespan.org

Diagnostic Inventory for Depression (DID)

INSTRUCTIONS: This questionnaire is about how you have been feeling <u>**during the past week**</u>. After each question there are 5 statements (numbered 0–4). Read all 5 statements carefully. Then decide which one best describes how you have been feeling. Choose only one statement per group. If more than one statement in a group applies to you, choose the one with the higher number.

(1) **During the past week, have you been feeling sad or depressed?**
0   No, not at all.
1   Yes, a little bit.
2   Yes, I have felt sad or depressed most of the time.
3   Yes, I have been very sad or depressed nearly all the time.
4   Yes, I have been extremely depressed nearly all the time.

(2) **How many days in the past 2 weeks have you been feeling sad or depressed?**
0   No days
1   A few days
2   About half the days
3   Nearly every day
4   Every day

(3) **Which of the following best describes your level of interest in your usual activities during the past week?**
0   I have not lost interest in my usual activities.
1   I have been less interested in 1 or 2 of my usual activities.
2   I have been less interested in several of my usual activities.
3   I have lost most of my interest in almost all of my usual activities.
4   I have lost all interest in all of my usual activities.

(4) **How many days in the past 2 weeks have you been less interested in your usual activities?**
0   No days
1   A few days
2   About half the days
3   Nearly every day
4   Every day

(5) **Which of the following best describes the amount of pleasure you have gotten from your usual activities during the past week?**
0   I have gotten as much pleasure as usual.
1   I have gotten a little less pleasure from 1 or 2 of my usual activities.
2   I have gotten less pleasure from several of my usual activities.
3   I have gotten almost no pleasure from most of the activities that I usually enjoy.
4   I have gotten no pleasure from any of the activities that I usually enjoy.

(6) **How many days in the past 2 weeks have you gotten less pleasure from your usual activities?**
0   No days
1   A few days
2   About half the days
3   Nearly every day
4   Every day

(7) **During the past week, has your energy level been low?**
0   No, not at all.
1   Yes, my energy level has occasionally been a little lower than it normally is.
2   Yes, I have clearly had less energy than I normally do.
3   Yes, I have had much less energy than I normally have.
4   Yes, I have felt exhausted almost all of the time.

(8) **Which of the following best describes your level of physical restlessness during the past week?**
0   I have not been more restless and fidgety than usual.
1   I have been a little more restless and fidgety than usual.

2   I have been very fidgety, and it has been somewhat difficult to sit still.
3   I have been extremely fidgety, and I have been pacing a little bit almost every day.
4   I have been pacing more than an hour a day, and I have been unable to sit still.

(9) **Which of the following best describes your physical activity level during the past week?**
0   I have not been moving more slowly than usual.
1   I have been moving a little more slowly than usual.
2   I have been moving more slowly than usual, and it takes me longer than usual to do most activities.
3   Normal activities are difficult because it has been tough to start moving.
4   I have been feeling extremely slowed down physically, like I am stuck in mud.

(10) **During the past week, have you been bothered by feelings of guilt?**
0   No, not at all.
1   Yes, I have occasionally felt a little guilty.
2   Yes, I have often been bothered by feelings of guilt.
3   Yes, I have often been bothered by strong feelings of guilt.
4   Yes, I have been feeling extremely guilty.

(11) **During the past week, what has your self esteem been like?**
0   My self-esteem has not been low.
1   Once in a while, my opinion of myself has been a little low.
2   I often think I am a failure.
3   I almost always think I am a failure.
4   I have been thinking I am a totally useless and worthless person.

(12) **During the past week, have you been thinking about death or dying?**
0   No, not at all.
1   Yes, I have occasionally thought that life is not worth living.
2   Yes, I have frequently thought about dying in passive ways (such as going to sleep and not waking up).
3   Yes, I have frequently thought about death, and that others would be better off if I were dead.
4   Yes, I have been wishing I were dead.

(13) **During the past week, have you been thinking about killing yourself?**
0   No, not at all.
1   Yes, I had a fleeting thought about killing myself.
2   Yes, several times I thought about killing myself, but I would not act on these thoughts.
3   Yes, I have been seriously thinking about killing myself.
4   Yes, I have thought of a specific plan for killing myself.

(14) **Which of the following best describes your ability to concentrate during the past week?**
0   I have been able to concentrate as well as usual.
1   My ability to concentrate has been slightly worse than usual.
2   My attention span has not been as good as usual and I have had difficulty collecting my thoughts, but this hasn't caused any serious problems.
3   I have frequently had trouble concentrating, and it has interfered with my usual activities.
4   It has been so hard to concentrate that even simple things are hard to do.

(15) **During the past week, have you had trouble making decisions?**

0   No, not at all.
1   Yes, making decisions has been slightly more difficult than usual.
2   Yes, it has been harder and has taken longer to make decisions, but I have been making them.
3   Yes, I have been unable to make some decisions that I would usually have been able to make.
4   Yes, important things are not getting done because I have had trouble making decisions.

(16) **During the past week, has your appetite been <u>decreased</u>?**

0   No, not at all.
1   Yes, my appetite has been slightly decreased compared to how it normally is.
2   Yes, my appetite has been clearly decreased, but I have been eating about as much as I normally do.
3   Yes, my appetite has been clearly decreased, and I have been eating less than I normally do.
4   Yes, my appetite has been very bad, and I have had to force myself to eat even a little.

(17) **How much weight have you <u>lost</u> during the past week (not due to dieting)?**

0   None (or the only weight I lost was due to dieting)
1   1–2 pounds
2   3–5 pounds
3   6–10 pounds
4   More than 10 pounds

(18) **During the past week, has your appetite been <u>increased</u>?**

0   No, not at all.
1   Yes, my appetite has been slightly increased compared to how it normally is.
2   Yes, my appetite has clearly been increased compared to how it normally is.
3   Yes, my appetite has been greatly increased compared to how it normally do.

4   Yes, I have been feeling hungry all the time.

(19) **How much weight have you <u>gained</u> during the past week?**

0   None
1   1–2 pounds
2   3–5 pounds
3   6–10 pounds
4   More than 10 pounds

(20) **During the past week, have you been sleeping <u>less</u> than you normally do?**

0   No, not at all.
1   Yes, I have occasionally had slight difficulty sleeping.
2   Yes, I have clearly been sleeping less than I normally do.
3   Yes, I have been sleeping about half my normal amount of time.
4   Yes, I have been sleeping less than 2 hours a night.

(21) **During the past week, have you been sleeping <u>more</u> than you normally do?**

0   No, not at all.
1   Yes, I have occasionally slept more than I normally do.
2   Yes, I have frequently slept at least 1 hour more than I normally do.
3   Yes, I have frequently slept at least 2 hours more than I normally do.
4   Yes, I have frequently slept at least 3 hours more than I normally do.

(22) **During the past week, have you been feeling pessimistic or hopeless about the future?**

0   No, not at all.
1   Yes, I have occasionally felt a little pessimistic about the future.
2   Yes, I have often felt pessimistic about the future.
3   Yes, I have been feeling very pessimistic about the future most of the time.
4   Yes, I have been feeling that there is no hope for the future.

---

0 = no difficulty   1 = mild difficulty   2 = moderate difficulty   3 = marked difficulty   4 = extreme difficulty

INSTRUCTIONS

Indicate below how much symptoms of depression have interfered with, or caused difficulties in, the following areas of your life during the past week. (Circle DNA [Does Not Apply] if you are not married or have a boyfriend/girlfriend.)

During the PAST WEEK, how much difficulty have symptoms of depression caused in your...

23. usual daily responsibilities (at a paid job, at home, or at school)		0	1	2	3	4
24. relationship with your husband, wife, boyfriend, girlfriend, or lover	DNA	0	1	2	3	4
25. relationships with close family members		0	1	2	3	4
26. relationships with your friends		0	1	2	3	4
27. participation and enjoyment in leisure and recreation activities		0	1	2	3	4

28. Overall, how much have symptoms of depression interfered with or caused difficulties in your life?

0) not at all
1) a little bit
2) a moderate amount
3) quite a bit
4) extremely

29. How many days during the past week were you <u>completely unable</u> to perform your usual daily responsibilities (at a paid job, at home, or at school) because you were feeling depressed? (circle one)

0 days   1 day   2 days   3 days   4 days   5 days   6 days   7 days

Diagnostic Inventory for Depression (DID) (continued)

0 = very satisfied   1 = mostly satisfied   2 = equally satisfied/dissatisfied   3 = mostly dissatisfied   4 = very dissatisfied

INSTRUCTIONS

Indicate below your level of satisfaction with the following areas of your life (Circle DNA [Does Not Apply] if you are not married or have a boyfriend or girlfriend.)

During the PAST WEEK how satisfied have you been with your...

30.	usual daily responsibilities (at a paid job, at home, or at school)		0	1	2	3	4
31.	relationship with your husband, wife, boyfriend, girlfriend, or lover	DNA	0	1	2	3	4
32.	relationship with close family members		0	1	2	3	4
33.	relationships with your friends		0	1	2	3	4
34.	participation and enjoyment in leisure and recreation activities		0	1	2	3	4
35.	mental health		0	1	2	3	4
36.	physical health		0	1	2	3	4

37. In general, how satisfied have you been with your life during the past week?
- 0) very satisfied
- 1) mostly satisfied
- 2) equally satisfied & dissatisfied
- 3) mostly dissatisfied
- 4) very dissatisfied

38. In general, how would you rate your overall quality of life during the past week?
- 0) very good, my life could hardly be better
- 1) pretty good, most things are going well
- 2) the good and bad parts are about equal
- 3) pretty bad, most things are going poorly
- 4) very bad, my life could hardly be worse

Reproduced from Zimmerman M, Sheeran T, Young D. J Clin Psychol 2004; 60(1):87–110. © 2004 Mark Zimmerman.

Hamilton Depression Inventory (HDI)

Reference: **Reynolds WM, Kobak KA. Hamilton Depression Inventory (HDI): Professional Manual. 1995. Odessa, FL, Psychological Assessment Resources**

Rating Self-report

Administration time 10–15 minutes

Main purpose To provide a self-report version of the HDRS

Population Adults

Commentary

The HDI is a 23-item self-report inventory that assesses depressive symptomatology for the previous 2 weeks. Developed as a patient-rated version of the Hamilton Depression Rating Scale (see page 28), the instrument reflects DSM-IV criteria and assesses both frequency and severity of depressive symptoms. A 17-item version (that parallels the 17-item clinician-rated HAM-D) and melancholia sub-scale can be derived, and a 9-item short-form version is available for use as a screening tool.

Scoring

Scoring varies by item, with a total range of 0–73, where higher scores indicate greater depression severity. A score of 19 has been suggested as a cut-off score when screening for depression.

Versions

The scale has been translated into Arabic, and a computer-administered version is available.

Additional reference

Dozois DJ. The psychometric characteristics of the Hamilton Depression Inventory. J Pers Assess 2003; 80(1):31–40.

Address for correspondence

Psychological Assessment Resources, Inc.
16204 N. Florida Avenue, Lutz, FL 33549, USA
Telephone: 1-800-331-8378 or 1-813-968-3003
Email: custserv@parinc.com
Website: www.parinc.com

Hamilton Depression Inventory (HDI) – sample items

How often do you cry or feel like crying?
0   Rarely
1   Slightly more than usual for me
2   Quite a bit more than usual for me
3   Nearly all the time

Do you feel helpless or incapable of getting everyday tasks done?
0   Not at all
1   Occasionally
2   Often
3   Almost constantly

Over the past 2 weeks, how often did you have difficulty making decisions?
0   Not at all or rarely
1   Occasionally
2   Often (about half of the time)
3   Very often
4   Almost all of the time

Hamilton Depression Rating Scale (HDRS)

Reference: **Hamilton M. A rating scale for depression. J Neurol Neurosurg Psychiatry 1960; 23:56–62**

Rating Clinician-rated

Administration time 20–30 minutes

Main purpose To assess severity of, and change in, depressive symptoms

Population Adults

Commentary

The HDRS (also known as the Ham-D) is the most widely used clinician-administered depression assessment scale. The original version contains 17 items (HDRS$_{17}$) pertaining to symptoms of depression experienced over the past week. Although the scale was designed for completion after an unstructured clinical interview, there are now semi-structured interview guides available. The HDRS was originally developed for hospital inpatients, thus the emphasis on melancholic and physical symptoms of depression. A later 21-item version (HDRS$_{21}$) included 4 items intended to subtype the depression, but which are sometimes, incorrectly, used to rate severity. A limitation of the HDRS is that atypical symptoms of depression (e.g., hypersomnia, hyperphagia) are not assessed (see SIGH-SAD, page 55).

Scoring

Method for scoring varies by version. For the HDRS$_{17}$, a score of 0–7 is generally accepted to be within the normal range (or in clinical remission), while a score of 20 or higher (indicating at least moderate severity) is usually required for entry into a clinical trial.

Versions

The scale has been translated into a number of languages including French, German, Italian, Thai, and Turkish. As well, there is an Interactive Voice Response version (IVR), a Seasonal Affective Disorder version (SIGH-SAD, see page 55), and a Structured Interview Version (HDS-SIV). Numerous versions with varying lengths include the HDRS17, HDRS21, HDRS29, HDRS8, HDRS6, HDRS24, and HDRS7 (see page 30).

Additional references

Hamilton M. Development of a rating scale for primary depressive illness. Br J Soc Clin Psychol 1967; 6(4):278–96.

Williams JB. A structured interview guide for the Hamilton Depression Rating Scale. Arch Gen Psychiatry 1988; 45(8):742–7.

Address for correspondence

The HDRS is in the public domain.

Hamilton Depression Rating Scale (HDRS)

Patient Name: _____

Date: (dd/mon/yr) _____ / _____ / _____

Rater: _____

1. Depressed Mood
- 0 Absent.
- 1 These feeling states indicated only on questioning.
- 2 These feeling states spontaneously reported verbally.
- 3 Communicates feeling states non-verbally – i.e., through facial expression, posture, voice, and tendency to weep.
- 4 Patient reports virtually only these feeling states in his spontaneous verbal and non-verbal communication.

2. Work and Activities
- 0 No difficulty.
- 1 Thoughts and feelings of incapacity, fatigue or weakness related to activities; work or hobbies.
- 2 Loss of interest in activities; hobbies or work – either directly reported by patient, or indirect in listlessness, indecision and vacillation (feels he has to push self to work or activities).
- 3 Decrease in actual time spent in activities or decrease in productivity. In hospital rate 3 if patient does not spend at least three hours a day in activities (hospital job or hobbies) exclusive of ward chores.
- 4 Stopped working because of present illness. In hospital, rate 4 if patient engages in no activities except ward chores, or if patient fails to perform ward chores unassisted.

3. Genital Symptoms
- 0 Absent.
- 1 Mild.
- 2 Severe.

4. Somatic Symptoms – GI
- 0 None.
- 1 Loss of appetite but eating without staff encouragement. Heavy feelings in abdomen.
- 2 Difficulty eating without staff urging. Requests or requires laxatives or medication for bowels or medication for G.I. symptoms.

5. Loss of Weight
- 0 No weight loss.
- 1 Probable weight loss associated with present illness.
- 2 Definite (according to patient) weight loss.

6. Insomnia – Early
- 0 No difficulty falling asleep.
- 1 Complains of occasional difficulty falling asleep – i.e., more than 1/2 hour.
- 2 Complains of nightly difficulty falling asleep.

7. Insomnia – Middle
- 0 No difficulty.
- 1 Patient complains of being restless and disturbed during the night.
- 2 Waking during the night – any getting out of bed rates 2 (except for purposes of voiding).

8. Insomnia – Late
- 0 No difficulty.
- 1 Waking in early hours of the morning but goes back to sleep.
- 2 Unable to fall asleep again if he gets out of bed.

9. Somatic Symptoms – General
- 0 None.
- 1 Heaviness in limbs, back or head. Backaches, headache, muscle aches. Loss of energy and fatigability.
- 2 Any clear-cut symptom rates 2.

10. Feelings of Guilt
- 0 Absent.
- 1 Self reproach, feels he has let people down.
- 2 Ideas of guilt or rumination over past errors or sinful deeds.
- 3 Present illness is a punishment. Delusions of guilt.
- 4 Hears accusatory or denunciatory voices and/or experiences threatening visual hallucinations.

11. Suicide
- 0 Absent.
- 1 Feels life is not worth living.
- 2 Wishes he were dead or any thoughts of possible death to self.
- 3 Suicide ideas or gestures.
- 4 Attempts at suicide (any serious attempt rates 4).

12. Anxiety – Psychic
- 0 No difficulty.
- 1 Subjective tension and irritability.
- 2 Worrying about minor matters.
- 3 Apprehensive attitude apparent in face or speech.
- 4 Fears expressed without questioning.

13. Anxiety – Somatic
- 0 Absent.
- 1 Mild.
- 2 Moderate.
- 3 Severe.
- 4 Incapacitating.

14. Hypochondriasis
- 0 Not present
- 1 Self-absorption (bodily).
- 2 Preoccupation with health.
- 3 Frequent complaints, requests for help, etc.
- 4 Hypochondriacal delusions.

15. Insight
- 0 Acknowledges being depressed and ill.
- 1 Acknowledges illness but attributes cause to bad food, climate, over work, virus, need for rest, etc.
- 2 Denies being ill at all.

16. Motor Retardation
- 0 Normal speech and thought.
- 1 Slight retardation at interview.
- 2 Obvious retardation at interview.
- 3 Interview difficult.
- 4 Complete stupor.

17. Agitation
- 0 None.
- 1 Fidgetiness.
- 2 Playing with hands, hair, etc.
- 3 Moving about can't sit still.
- 4 Hand wringing, nail biting, hair pulling, biting of lips.

17-item HAMD Total: _____

Reproduced from Hamilton M. J Neurol Neurosurg Psychiatry 1960; 23:56–62,

Hamilton Depression Rating Scale, 7-item version (HAM-D7)

Reference: **McIntyre R, Kennedy S, Bagby RM, Bakish D. Assessing full remission. J Psychiatry Neurosci 2002; 27(4):235–9**

Rating Clinician-rated

Administration time 7–10 minutes

Main purpose To assess severity of, and change in, depressive symptoms

Population Adults

Commentary

This abbreviated version of the 17-item HDRS (see page 28) was developed for use in primary care settings where interviewing time is limited. The HAM-D7, also referred to as the Toronto HAM-D7, performs as well as the HDRS and the MADRS (see page 40) in tracking change over time.

Scoring

A score of 0–3 indicates clinical remission, equivalent to a score of 0–7 on the HDRS.

Versions

No other versions of the HAM-D7 are currently available.

Additional reference

McIntyre RS, Fulton KA, Bakish D, Jordan J, Kennedy SH. The HAM-D7: A brief depression scale to distinguish antidepressant response from symptomatic remission. Primary Psychiatry 2003; 10(1): 39–42.

Address for correspondence

Dr. R. Michael Bagby
Director, Clinical Research Department
Centre for Addiction and Mental Health
250 College St., Toronto ON, M5T 1R8, Canada
Telephone: 1-416-535-8501 ext. 6939
Email: michael_bagby@camh.net

Hamilton Depression Rating Scale, 7-item version (HAM-D7)

Patient Name: _____

Rater: _____

Date: (dd/mon/yr) _____ / _____ / _____

1   Depressed Mood
  0   Absent.
  1   These feeling states indicated only on questioning.
  2   These feeling states spontaneously reported verbally.
  3   Communicates feeling states non-verbally – i.e., through facial expression, posture, voice, and tendency to weep.
  4   Patient reports virtually only these feeling states in his spontaneous verbal and non-verbal communication.

2   Feelings of Guilt
  0   Absent.
  1   Self reproach, feels he has let people down.
  2   Ideas of guilt or rumination over past errors or sinful deeds.
  3   Present illness is a punishment. Delusions of guilt.
  4   Hears accusatory or denunciatory voices and/or experiences threatening visual hallucinations.

3   Suicide
  0   Absent.
  1   Feels life is not worth living.
  2   Wishes he were dead or any thoughts of possible death to self.
  3   Suicide ideas or gestures.
  4   Attempts at suicide (any serious attempt rates 4).

4   Work and Activities
  0   No difficulty.
  1   Thoughts and feelings of incapacity, fatigue or weakness related to activities; work or hobbies.

  2   Loss of interest in activities; hobbies or work – either directly reported by patient, or indirect in listlessness, indecision and vacillation (feels he has to push self to work or activities).
  3   Decrease in actual time spent in activities or decrease in productivity. In hospital rate 3 if patient does not spend at least three hours a day in activities (hospital job or hobbies) exclusive of ward chores.
  4   Stopped working because of present illness. In hospital, rate 4 if patient engages in no activities except ward chores, or if patient fails to perform ward chores unassisted.

5   Anxiety – Psychic
  0   No difficulty.
  1   Subjective tension and irritability.
  2   Worrying about minor matters.
  3   Apprehensive attitude apparent in face or speech.
  4   Fears expressed without questioning.

6   Anxiety – Somatic
  0   Absent.
  1   Mild.
  2   Moderate.
  3   Severe.
  4   Incapacitating.

7   Somatic Symptoms – General
  0   None.
  1   Heaviness in limbs, back or head. Backaches, headache, muscle aches. Loss of energy and fatigability.
  2   Any clear-cut symptom rates 2.

7-item HAMD total: _____

The intellectual property rights for the mathematical algorithm used to design this scale reside with Dr. Michael Bagby and the Center for Addiction and Mental Health.

Harvard National Depression Screening Scale (HANDS)

Reference: **Baer L, Jacobs DG, Meszler-Reizes J, Blais M, Fava M, Kessler R, Magruder K, Murphy J, Kopans B, Cukor P, Leahy L, O'Laughlen J. Development of a brief screening instrument: the HANDS. Psychother Psychosom 2000; 69(1):35–41**

Rating Self-report

Administration time 10 minutes

Main purpose To screen for major depressive disorder

Population Adults

Commentary

The HANDS was developed as a brief, easy-to-score self-report depression screening tool for use in the National Depression Screening Day initiative. A 10-item questionnaire, the HANDS assesses occurrence of depressive symptoms over the previous two weeks. Research has indicated that this brief measure performs as well as the 20-item Zung Self-Rating Depression Scale (see page 59) and the Beck Depression Inventory–II (see page 10).

Scoring

To select potential cases of depression, a cut-off score of 9 is recommended by the scale's developers.

Versions

No other versions are currently available.

Additional references

None available.

Address for correspondence

Screening for Mental Health, Inc.
One Washington Street, Suite 304
Wellesley Hills, MA 02481-1706, USA
Telephone: 1-781-239-0071
Website: www.mentalhealthscreening.org

HANDS Depression Screening Tool

Over the <u>past two weeks</u>, how often have you:	None or little of the time	Some of the time	Most of the time	All of the time
1. been feeling low in energy, slowed down?	☐	☐	☐	☐
2. been blaming yourself for things?	☐	☐	☐	☐
3. had poor appetite?	☐	☐	☐	☐
4. had difficulty falling asleep, staying asleep?	☐	☐	☐	☐
5. been feeling hopeless about the future?	☐	☐	☐	☐
6. been feeling blue?	☐	☐	☐	☐
7. been feeling no interest in things?	☐	☐	☐	☐
8. had feelings of worthlessness?	☐	☐	☐	☐
9. thought about or wanted to commit suicide?	☐	☐	☐	☐
10. had difficulty concentrating or making decisions?	☐	☐	☐	☐

Inventory of Depressive Symptomatology (IDS)

Reference: **Rush AJ, Gullion CM, Basco MR, Jarrett RB, Trivedi MH. The Inventory of Depressive Symptomatology (IDS): psychometric properties. Psychol Med 1996; 26(3):477–86**

Rating Self-report (IDS-SR) or clinician-rated (IDS-C)

Administration time IDS-SR (10–15 minutes) or IDS-C (15–20 minutes); QIDS-SR or QIDS-C <10 minutes

Main purpose To assess severity of, and change in, depressive symptoms

Population Adults, adolescents and older adults

Commentary

The 30-item IDS is available in either self-report (IDS-SR) or clinician-rated (IDS-C) formats. Asking respondents to rate how they have felt over the past week, both versions of the IDS assesses frequency, duration or severity of a wide range of depressive symptoms. Both versions of the scale assess all 9 symptom domains needed to diagnose a DSM-IV major depressive episode in order to assess for symptom remission and include items to assess melancholic, and atypical symptom features as well as commonly associated symptoms such as anxiety or pain. The instruments are scaled to allow the detection of milder levels of depression, exclude uncommonly encountered items (e.g. depersonalization) and do not rate psychotic symptoms. The 30-item versions of the IDS take approximately 15–20 minutes to administer, however, and may be too time-consuming for many clinicians. Consequently, a briefer version of the scale, the 16-item Quick Inventory of Depressive Symptomatology (QIDS), has been developed in both self-report and clinician-rated versions. The patient rated QIDS appears to be as sensitive to symptom change as the IDS-SR and takes only 5–10 minutes to administer. The QIDS-SR is reproduced in full here.

Scoring

Items on the IDS-SR are scored on a 0–3 scale, although respondents answer EITHER question 11 or 12 (decreased appetite or increased appetite) and EITHER question 13 or 14 (weight loss or weight gain). Consequently, the total score range for the 30-item version is 0–84, with higher scores denoting greater symptom severity. The authors suggest the following severity indications for the 30-item IDS-C: ≤12, normal; 13–23, mild; 24–36, moderate; 37–46 moderate-severe; ≥47 severe. For the 30-item IDS-SR (total score range 0–24): ≤14, normal; 15–25, mild; 26–38, moderate; 39–48, moderate-severe; ≥49, severe. For the QIDS-C and QIDS-SR: ≤5, normal; 6–10, mild; 11–15, moderate; 16–20, severe; ≥21, very severe.

Versions

Both the IDS and the QIDS have been translated into a variety of languages, including: Chinese, Danish, Dutch, French, German, Italian, Norwegian, Portuguese, Spanish and Turkish (see http://www.star-d.org). Both the IDS and QIDS are available in English (and the QIDS in Spanish) in an Interactive Voice Response (IVR) system (Healthcare Technology Systems, Madison, Wisconsin). All paper versions of these instruments are in the public domain and may be used without permission.

Additional references

Corruble E, Legrand JM, Duret C, Charles G, Guelfi JD. IDS-C and IDS-SR: psychometric properties in depressed in-patients. J Affect Disord 1999; 56(2–3):95–101.

Rush AJ, Trivedi MH, Ibrahim HM, Carmody TJ, Arnow B, Klein DN, Markowitz JC, Ninan PT, Kornstein S, Manber R, Thase ME, Kocsis JH, Keller MB. The 16-Item Quick Inventory of Depressive Symptomatology (QIDS), Clinician Rating (QIDS-C), and Self-Report (QIDS-SR): a psychometric evaluation in patients with chronic major depression. Biol Psychiatry 2003; 54(5):573–83.

Trivedi MH, Rush AJ, Ibrahim HM, Carmody TJ, Biggs MM, Suppes T, Crismon ML, Shores-Wilson K, Toprac MG, Dennehy EB, Witte B, Kashner TM. The Inventory of Depressive Symptomatology, Clinician Rating (IDS-C) and Self-Report (IDS-SR), and the Quick Inventory of Depressive Symptomatology, Clinical Rating (QIDS-C) and Self-Report (QIDS-SR) in public sector patients with mood disorders, A psychometric evaluation. Psychol Med 2004; 34(1):73–82.

Address for correspondence

Dr. A. John Rush
Department of Psychiatry
University of Texas Southwestern Medical Center
5323 Harry Hines Blvd., Dallas, TX 75390–9086, USA
Telephone: 1-214-648-4600
Email: john.rush@utsouthwestern.edu

Quick Inventory of Depressive Symptomatology (Self-Report) (QIDS-SR)

Name _____   Today's date _____

Please circle the one response to each item that best describes you for the past seven days.

1.   Falling Asleep
 0   I never take longer than 30 minutes to fall asleep.
 1   I take at least 30 minutes to fall asleep, less than half the time.
 2   I take at least 30 minutes to fall asleep, more than half the time.
 3   I take more than 60 minutes to fall asleep, more than half the time.

2.   Sleep During the Night
 0   I do not wake up at night.
 1   I have a restless, light sleep with a few brief awakenings each night.
 2   I wake up at least once a night, but I go back to sleep easily.
 3   I awaken more than once a night and stay awake for 20 minutes or more, more than half the time.

3.   Waking Up Too Early
 0   Most of the time, I awaken no more than 30 minutes before I need to get up.
 1   More than half the time, I awaken more than 30 minutes before I need to get up.
 2   I almost always awaken at least one hour or so before I need to, but I go back to sleep eventually.
 3   I awaken at least one hour before I need to, and can't go back to sleep.

4.   Sleeping Too Much
 0   I sleep no longer than 7–8 hours/night, without napping during the day.
 1   I sleep no longer than 10 hours in a 24-hour period including naps.
 2   I sleep no longer than 12 hours in a 24-hour period including naps.
 3   I sleep longer than 12 hours in a 24-hour period including naps.

5.   Feeling Sad
 0   I do not feel sad.
 1   I feel sad less than half the time.
 2   I feel sad more than half the time.
 3   I feel sad nearly all of the time.

6.   Decreased Appetite
 0   There is no change in my usual appetite.
 1   I eat somewhat less often or lesser amounts of food than usual.
 2   I eat much less than usual and only with personal effort.
 3   I rarely eat within a 24-hour period, and only with extreme personal effort or when others persuade me to eat.

7.   Increased Appetite
 0   There is no change from my usual appetite.
 1   I feel a need to eat more frequently than usual.
 2   I regularly eat more often and/or greater amounts of food than usual.
 3   I feel driven to overeat both at mealtime and between meals.

8.   Decreased Weight (Within the Last Two Weeks)
 0   I have not had a change in my weight.
 1   I feel as if I've had a slight weight loss.
 2   I have lost 2 pounds or more.
 3   I have lost 5 pounds or more.

9.   Increased Weight (Within the Last Two Weeks)
 0   I have not had a change in my weight.
 1   I feel as if I've had a slight weight gain.
 2   I have gained 2 pounds or more.
 3   I have gained 5 pounds or more.

10.   Concentration/Decision Making
 0   There is no change in my usual capacity to concentrate or make decisions.
 1   I occasionally feel indecisive or find that my attention wanders.
 2   Most of the time, I struggle to focus my attention or to make decisions.
 3   I cannot concentrate well enough to read or cannot make even minor decisions.

11.   View of Myself
 0   I see myself as equally worthwhile and deserving as other people.
 1   I am more self-blaming than usual.
 2   I largely believe that I cause problems for others.
 3   I think almost constantly about major and minor defects in myself.

12. **Thoughts of Death or Suicide**
    0   I do not think of suicide or death.
    1   I feel that life is empty or wonder if it's worth living.
    2   I think of suicide or death several times a week for several minutes.
    3   I think of suicide or death several times a day in some detail, or I have made specific plans for suicide or have actually tried to take my life.

13. **General Interest**
    0   There is no change from usual in how interested I am in other people or activities.
    1   I notice that I am less interested in people or activities.
    2   I find I have interest in only one or two of my formerly pursued activities.
    3   I have virtually no interest in formerly pursued activities.

14. **Energy Level**
    0   There is no change in my usual level of energy.
    1   I get tired more easily than usual.
    2   I have to make a big effort to start or finish my usual daily activities (for example, shopping, homework, cooking or going to work).
    3   I really cannot carry out most of my usual daily activities because I just don't have the energy.

15. **Feeling slowed down**
    0   I think, speak, and move at my usual rate of speed.
    1   I find that my thinking is slowed down or my voice sounds dull or flat.
    2   It takes me several seconds to respond to most questions and I'm sure my thinking is slowed.
    3   I am often unable to respond to questions without extreme effort.

16. **Feeling restless**
    0   I do not feel restless.
    1   I'm often fidgety, wringing my hands, or need to shift how I am sitting.
    2   I have impulses to move about and am quite restless.
    3   At times, I am unable to stay seated and need to pace around.

To Score
1. Enter the highest score on any 1 of the 4 sleep items (1-4)   _____
2. Item 5   _____
3. Enter the highest score on any 1 appetite/weight item (6-9)   _____
4. Item 10   _____
5. Item 11   _____
6. Item 12   _____
7. Item 13   _____
8. Item 14   _____
9. Enter the highest score on either of the 2 psychomotor items (15 and 16)   _____

TOTAL SCORE (Range 0–27)   _____

Scoring Criteria
0–5   Normal
6–10   Mild
11–15   Moderate
16–20   Severe
≥21   Very Severe

This scale is in the public domain and can be reproduced without permission.

Manic State Rating Scale (MSRS)

Reference: Beigel A, Murphy DL, Bunney WE Jr. The manic-state rating scale: Scale construction, reliability, and validity. Arch Gen Psych 1971; 25:256–62

Rating Clinician-rated

Administration time 15 minutes

Main purpose To asses severity of manic symptoms

Population Adults

Commentary

The MSRS (also referred to as the Beigel scale) is a 26-item clinician-administered scale developed to assess severity of symptoms of mania. Relying upon observation of the patient rather than patient report, the MSRS is useful in situations where conducting an interview is difficult. However, the scale does not possess any anchor points, which may result in decreased inter-rater reliability, and is not widely used in clinical settings at the present time.

Scoring

Items are rated on a frequency (0–5 scale, range 0–130) and severity scale (1–5 scale, range 26–130), with higher scores indicating greater severity of manic symptoms.

Versions

A 28-item version (the Modified Manic State, Blackburn et al. 1977) is also available.

Additional references

Bech P, Bolwig TG, Dein E, Jacobsen O, Gram LF. Quantitative rating of manic states. Correlation between clinical assessment and Biegel's Objective Rating Scale. Acta Psychiatr Scand 1975; 52(1):1–6.

Blackburn IM, Loudon JB, Ashworth CM. A new scale for measuring mania. Psychol Med 1977; 7(3):453–8.

Lerer B, Moore N, Meyendorff E, Cho SR, Gershon S. Carbamazepine versus lithium in mania: a double-blind study. J Clin Psychiatry 1987; 48(3):89–93.

Address for correspondence

None available. The scale is in the public domain.

The Manic State Rating Scale

Part A Frequency (How much of the time?)						The Patient	Part B Intensity (How intense is it?)				
None	Infrequent	Some	Much	Most	All		Very minimal	Minimal	Moderate	Marked	Very marked
0	1	2	3	4	5		1	2	3	4	5
						1. Looks depressed					
						2. Is talking					
						3. Moves from one place to another					
						4. Makes threats					
						5. Has poor judgement					
						6. Dresses inappropriately					
						7. Looks happy and cheerful					
						8. Seeks out others					
						9. Is distractible					
						10. Has grandiose ideas					
						11. Is irritable					
						12. Is combative or destructive					
						13. Is delusional					
						14. Verbalizes depressive feelings					
						15. Is active					
						16. Is argumentative					
						17. Talks about sex					
						18. Is angry					
						19. Is careless about dress and grooming					
						20. Has diminished impulse control					
						21. Verbalizes feelings of well-being					
						22. Is suspicious					
						23. Makes unrealistic plans					
						24. Demands contact with others					
						25. Is sexually preoccupied					
						26. Jumps from one subject to another					

Reproduced from Beigel A, Murphy DL, Bunney WE Jr. Arch Gen Psych 1971; 25:256–62.

Medical Outcomes Study Depression Questionnaire

Reference: **Burnam MA, Wells KB, Leake B, Landsverk J. Development of a brief screening instrument for detecting depressive disorders. Med Care 1988; 26(8):775–89**

Rating Self-report

Administration time <5 minutes

Main purpose To screen for depression and dysthymia

Population Adults under 60 years

Commentary

The Medical Outcomes Study Depression Questionnaire is a brief screening tool designed to detect the presence of either MDD or dysthymia. The scale includes items taken from the 12-month Composite International Diagnostic Interview (CIDI) and questions assessing depressive symptoms over various time-frames.

Scoring

Items are scored in a yes/no format. A positive screen is indicated if the patient answers yes to questions 1 AND 1a and 1b, OR 2a or 2b, AND 3a or 3b.

Versions

The scale has been translated into Spanish.

Additional references

Nagel R, Lynch D, Tamburrino M. Validity of the medical outcomes study depression screener in family practice training centers and community settings. Fam Med 1998; 30(5):362–5.

Rumsfeld JS, Havranek E, Masoudi FA, Peterson ED, Jones P, Tooley JF, Krumholz HM, Spertus JA. Cardiovascular Outcomes Research Consortium. Depressive symptoms are the strongest predictors of short-term declines in health status in patients with heart failure. J Am Coll Cardiol 2003; 42(10):1811–17.

Address for correspondence

RAND Health Communications
1700 Main Street
P.O. Box 2138
Santa Monica, CA 90407-2138, USA
Telephone: 1-310-393-0411, ext. 7775
Website: www.rand.org/health

Medical Outcomes Study Depression Questionnaire

Almost everyone has experienced times of feeling sad or depressed, like when suffering from a severe illness, when a person close to you has died, or if there are problems at work or in the family. The following questions are about such times.

1. Have you ever had <u>2 years or more</u> in your life when you felt depressed or sad most days, even if you felt OK sometimes? (Circle one)

   Yes   No (Skip to Question 2)

a. Did any period like that ever last 2 years without an interruption of 2 full months when you felt OK?

   Yes   No (Skip to Question 2)

b. Did any of those long periods of feeling sad or depressed continue into the last 12 months?

   Yes   No

2. In the last <u>12 months</u>, have you had <u>2 weeks or longer</u> when ... (Circle one answer on each line)

a. nearly every day you felt sad, empty or depressed for most of the day?

   Yes   No

b. you lost interest in most things like work, hobbies, and other things you usually enjoyed?

   Yes   No

3. In the <u>last month</u> did you have a period of <u>I week or more</u> when ... (Circle one answer on each line)

a. nearly every day you felt sad, empty or depressed for most of the day?

   Yes   No

b. you lost interest in most things like work, hobbies, and other things you usually enjoyed?

   Yes   No

Check if

☐

I AND Ia and Ib are yes
OR
2a OR 2b is yes

AND

3a or 3b is yes

Montgomery–Asberg Depression Rating Scale (MADRS)

Reference: **Montgomery SA, Asberg M. A new depression scale designed to be sensitive to change. Br J Psychiatry 1979; 134:382–9**

Rating Clinician-rated

Administration time 5–10 minutes

Main purpose To assess depressive symptomatology, particularly change following treatment with antidepressant medication

Population Adults taking antidepressant medication

Commentary

The MADRS consists of 10 items, 9 of which are based upon patient report, with one additional item that requires the rater to assess the patient's apparent (observed) sadness. The MADRS is probably second only to the HDRS (see page 28) as the most frequently used scale to monitor change in response to treatment in pharmaceutical trials. The MADRS can be used 'for any time interval between ratings, be it weekly or otherwise, but this must be recorded'. The MADRS places greater emphasis upon psychological symptoms of depression (i.e. sadness, tension, lassitude, pessimistic thoughts, and suicidal thoughts) than somatic in comparison to other clinician-rated scales such as the HDRS.

Scoring

Items are rated on a 0–6 scale, yielding a total possible score of 60, where higher scores indicate greater depressive symptomatology. A score of ≤10 has been suggested as a remission criterion.

Versions

A patient-rated version (the MADRS-S) has been developed.

Additional references

Svanborg P, Asberg M. A comparison between the Beck Depression Inventory (BDI) and the self-rating version of the Montgomery–Asberg Depression Rating Scale (MADRS). J Affect Disord 2001; 64(2–3):203–16.

Hawley CJ, Gale TM, Sivakumaran T; Hertfordshire Neuroscience Research group. Defining remission by cut off score on the MADRS: selecting the optimal value. J Affect Disord 2002; 72(2):177–84.

Address for correspondence

Dr. Marie Asberg
Department of Clinical Neuroscience
Karolinska Institutet
Karolinska sjukhuset, 171 76 Stockholm, Sweden
Telephone: 08 517 744 20
Email: marie.asberg@ks.se

Montgomery–Asberg Depression Rating Scale (MADRS)

The rating should be based on a clinical interview moving from broadly phrased questions about symptoms to more detailed ones which allow a precise rating of severity. The rater must decide whether the rating lies on the defined scale steps (0, 2, 4, 6) or between them (1, 3, 5).

It is important to remember that it is only on rare occasions that a depressed patient is encountered who cannot be rated on the items in the scale. If definite answers cannot be elicited from the patient all relevant clues as well as information from other sources should be used as a basis for the rating in line with customary clinical practice.

The scale may be used for any time interval between ratings, be it weekly or otherwise but this must be recorded.

Item List
1. Apparent sadness
2. Reported sadness
3. Inner tension
4. Reduced sleep
5. Reduced appetite
6. Concentration difficulties
7. Lassitude
8. Inability to feel
9. Pessimistic thoughts
10. Suicidal thoughts

1. Apparent Sadness
Representing despondency, gloom and despair (more than just ordinary transient low spirits), reflected in speech, facial expression, and posture. Rated by depth and inability to brighten up.
- 0 No sadness.
- 1
- 2 Looks dispirited but does brighten up without difficulty.
- 3
- 4 Appears sad and unhappy most of the time.
- 5
- 6 Looks miserable all the time. Extremely despondent.

2. Reported sadness
Representing reports of depressed mood, regardless of whether it is reflected in appearance or not. Includes low spirits, despondency or the feeling of being beyond help and without hope.

Rate according to intensity, duration and the extent to which the mood is reported to be influenced by events.
- 0 Occasional sadness in keeping with the circumstances.
- 1
- 2 Sad or low but brightens up without difficulty.
- 3
- 4 Pervasive feelings of sadness or gloominess. The mood is still influenced by external circumstances.
- 5
- 6 Continuous or unvarying sadness, misery or despondency.

3. Inner tension
Representing feeling of ill-defined discomfort, edginess, inner turmoil, mental tension mounting to either panic, dread or anguish.

Rate according to intensity, frequency, duration and the extent of reassurance called for.
- 0 Placid. Only fleeting inner tension.
- 1
- 2 Occasional feelings of edginess and ill-defined discomfort.
- 3
- 4 Continuous feelings of inner tension or intermittent panic which the patient can only master with some difficulty.

- 5
- 6 Unrelenting dread or anguish. Overwhelming panic.

4. Reduced sleep
Representing the experience of reduced duration or depth of sleep compared to the subject's own normal pattern when well.
- 0 Sleeps as usual.
- 1
- 2 Slight difficulty dropping off to sleep or slightly reduced, light or fitful sleep.
- 3
- 4 Sleep reduced or broken by at least two hours.
- 5
- 6 Less than two or three hours sleep.

5. Reduced appetite
Representing the feeling of a loss of appetite compared with when well. Rate by loss of desire for food or the need to force oneself to eat.
- 0 Normal or increased appetite.
- 1
- 2 Slightly reduced appetite.
- 3
- 4 No appetite. Food is tasteless.
- 5
- 6 Needs persuasion to eat at all.

6. Concentration difficulties
Representing difficulties in collecting one's thoughts mounting to incapacitating lack of concentration. Rate according to intensity, frequency, and degree of incapacity produced.
- 0 No difficulties in concentrating.
- 1
- 2 Occasional difficulties in collecting one's thoughts.
- 3
- 4 Difficulties in concentration and sustaining thought which reduces ability to read or hold a conversation.
- 5
- 6 Unable to read or converse without great difficulty.

7. Lassitude
Representing a difficulty getting started or slowness initiating and performing everyday activities.
- 0 Hardly any difficulty in getting started. No sluggishness.
- 1
- 2 Difficulties in starting activities.
- 3
- 4 Difficulties in starting simple routine activities which are carried out with effort.
- 5
- 6 Complete lassitude. Unable to do anything without help.

8. Inability to feel
Representing the subjective experience of reduced interest in the surroundings, or activities that normally give pleasure. The ability to react with adequate emotion to circumstances or people is reduced.
- 0 Normal interest in the surroundings and in other people.
- 1
- 2 Reduced ability to enjoy usual interests.
- 3
- 4 Loss of interest in the surroundings. Loss of feelings for friends and acquaintances.
- 5
- 6 The experience of being emotionally paralyzed, inability to feel anger, grief or pleasure and a complete or even painful failure to feel for close relatives and friends.

9. **Pessimistic thoughts**
Representing thoughts of guilt, inferiority, self-reproach, sinfulness, remorse and ruin.
0   No pessimistic thoughts.
1
2   Fluctuating ideas of failure, self-reproach or self-depreciation.
3
4   Persistent self-accusations, or definite but still rational ideas of guilt or sin. Increasingly pessimistic about the future.
5
6   Delusions of ruin, remorse or unredeemable sin. Self-accusations, which are absurd and unshakable.

10. **Suicidal thoughts**
Representing the feeling that life is not worth living, that a natural death would be welcome, suicidal thoughts and preparations for suicide. Suicidal attempts should not in themselves influence the rating.
0   Enjoy life or takes it as it comes.
1
2   Weary of life. Only fleeting suicidal thoughts.
3
4   Probably better off dead. Suicidal thoughts are common and suicide is considered as a possible solution but without specific plans or intention.
5
6   Explicit plans for suicide when there is an opportunity. Active preparations for suicide.

Reproduced from Montgomery SA, Asberg M. Br J Psychiatry 1979; 134:382–9 with permission from the Royal College of Psychiatrists.

Mood Disorders Questionnaire (MDQ)

Reference: **Hirschfeld RM, Williams JB, Spitzer RL, Calabrese JR, Flynn L, Keck PE, Jr, Lewis L, McElroy SL, Post RM, Rapport DJ, Russell JM, Sachs GS, Zajecka J. Development and validation of a screening instrument for bipolar spectrum disorder: the Mood Disorder Questionnaire. Am J Psychiatry 2000; 157(11):1873–5**

Rating Self-report

Administration time 5–10 minutes

Main purpose To screen for bipolar spectrum disorders

Population Adults

Commentary

Bipolar spectrum disorders, particularly bipolar disorder type II, are under-diagnosed in primary care and psychiatric patient populations. The MDQ is a brief 13-item self-report questionnaire designed to screen for bipolar spectrum disorders (BD type I, II, cyclothymia and BD not otherwise specified). In a yes/no format, the scale screens for lifetime history of DSM-IV mania/hypomania. The MDQ is an easy-to-administer screening tool with good psychometric properties and high clinical utility.

Scoring

The screen is considered positive when 7 or more symptoms have occurred, several within the same time period, causing moderate to severe problems.

Versions

The scale has been translated into Finnish.

Additional references

Hirschfeld RM. The Mood Disorder Questionnaire: A simple, patient-rated screening instrument for bipolar disorder. Primary Care Companion. J Clin Psychiatry 2002; 4(1):9–11.

Hirschfeld RM, Calabrese JR, Weissman MM, Reed M, Davies MA, Frye MA, Keck PE Jr, Lewis L, McElroy SL, McNulty JP, Wagner KD. Screening for bipolar disorder in the community. J Clin Psychiatry 2003; 64(1):53–9.

Isometsa E, Suominen K, Mantere O, Valtonen H, Leppamaki S, Pippingskold M, Arvilommi P. The mood disorder questionnaire improves recognition of bipolar disorder in psychiatric care. BMC Psychiatry 2003; 3(1):8.

Address for correspondence

Dr. Robert M.A. Hirschfeld
Department of Psychiatry and Behavioural Sciences
University of Texas Medical Branch
1.302 Rebecca Sealy, 301 University Boulevard
Galveston, TX 77555-0188, USA
Telephone: 1-409-747-9791
Email: rohirsch@utmb.edu

Mood Disorders Questionnaire

1) Has there ever been a period of time when you were not your usual self and....   Yes   No

    you felt so good or so hyper that other people thought that you were not your normal self or you were so hyper you got into trouble?   ____   ____

    you were so irritable that you shouted at people or started fights or arguments?   ____   ____

    you felt much more self-confident than usual?   ____   ____

    you got much less sleep than usual and found you didn't really miss it?   ____   ____

    you were much more talkative or spoke faster than usual?   ____   ____

    thoughts raced through your head or you couldn't slow your mind down?   ____   ____

    you were so easily distracted by things around you that you had trouble concentrating or staying on track?   ____   ____

    you had much more energy than usual?   ____   ____

    you were much more active or did many more things than usual?   ____   ____

    you were much more social or outgoing than usual, for example, you telephone friends in the middle of the night?   ____   ____

    you were much more interested in sex than usual?   ____   ____

    you did things that were unusual for you or that other people might have thought were excessive, foolish, or risky?   ____   ____

    spending money got you or your family into trouble?   ____   ____

2) If you checked YES to more than one of the above, have several of these ever happened during the same period of time? Please circle one response only.   **YES   NO**

3) How much of a problem did any of these cause you – like being unable to work; having family, money, or legal troubles; getting into arguments or fights? *Please circle one response only.*

No problem   Minor problem   Moderate problem   Serious problem

Diagnosis of hypomania is positive if: **7 or more** items endorsed in Q.I, plus **YES** for Q.2, plus **MODERATE or SERIOUS** problem for Q.3.

Reproduced from Hirschfeld RM, Williams JB, Spitzer RL, et al. Am J Psychiatry 2000; 157(11):1873–5.
© 2000 Robert Hirschfeld.

Patient Health Questionnaire 9 (PHQ-9)

Reference: Kroenke K, Spitzer RL, Williams JB. The PHQ-9: validity of a brief depression severity measure. J Gen Intern Med 2001; 16(9):606–13

Rating Self-report

Administration time <5 minutes

Main purpose To screen for depression in primary care

Population Adults and adolescents

Commentary

The PHQ-9 represents the depression sub-scale of the full version of the Patient Health Questionnaire (see page 145). A 9-item self-report scale designed to screen for depression in primary care, the instrument assesses depressive symptoms as defined by DSM-IV over the previous 2 weeks, and contains one question concerning functional impairment. The scale is appropriate for use both as a screening tool, and to monitor change over time. In a recent study, the PHQ-9 was shown to have superior psychometric properties than the Hospital Anxiety and Depression Scale (see page 81) and the Well Being Index (WBI-5, not reviewed here) in identifying major depressive disorder (Lowe et al., 2004).

Scoring

Items 1–9 are scored on a 0–3 scale, item 10 (functional status) is scored on a 4-point scale, ranging from 'not difficult at all' through to 'extremely difficult'. Full scoring methods are described in the Quick Guide to PRIME-MD Patient Health Questionnaire (PHQ) document (available from authors). Scores ranging between 1–4 indicate minimal depression, 5–9 mild depression, 10–14, moderate depression, 15–19, moderately severe depression, 20–27, severe depression.

Versions

The scale has been translated into Chinese, French, German, Greek, Italian, Spanish and Vietnamese.

Additional references

Kroenke K, Spitzer RL. The PHQ-9: A new depression and diagnostic severity measure. Psychiatr Ann 2002; 32:509–21.

Kroenke K, Spitzer RL, Williams JB. The Patient Health Questionnaire-2: validity of a two-item depression screener. Med Care 2003; 41(11):1284–92.

Lowe B, Spitzer RL, Grafe K, Kroenke K, Quenter A, Zipfel S, Buchholz C, Witte S, Herzog W. Comparative validity of three screening questionnaires for DSM-IV depressive disorders and physicians' diagnoses. J Affect Disord 2004; 78(2):131–40.

Address for correspondence

Dr. Robert L. Spitzer
Columbia University
1051 Riverside Drive, Unit 60
NYS Psychiatric Institute
New York, NY 10032, USA
Telephone: 1-212-543-5524
Email: RLS8@Columbia.edu

The PHQ is a trademark of Pfizer Inc.

Patient Health Questionnaire – PHQ-9 (www.primary-care.org)

Patient name: _____ Date: _____

1. Over the last 2 weeks, how often have you been bothered by any of the following problems?

	Not at all (0)	Several days(1)	More than half the days (2)	Nearly every day (3)
a. Little interest or pleasure in doing things.	☐	☐	☐	☐
b. Feeling down, depressed, or hopeless.	☐	☐	☐	☐
c. Trouble falling/staying asleep, sleeping too much.	☐	☐	☐	☐
d. Feeling tired or having little energy.	☐	☐	☐	☐
e. Poor appetite or overeating.	☐	☐	☐	☐
f. Feeling bad about yourself, or that you are a failure, or have let yourself or your family down.	☐	☐	☐	☐
g. Trouble concentrating on things, such as reading the newspaper or watching TV.	☐	☐	☐	☐
h. Moving or speaking so slowly that other people could have noticed. Or the opposite; being so fidgety or restless that you have been moving around more than usual.	☐	☐	☐	☐
i. Thoughts that you would be better off dead or of hurting yourself in some way.	☐	☐	☐	☐

2. If you checked off any problem on this questionnaire so far, how difficult have these problems made it for you to do your work, take care of things at home, or get along with other people?

☐ Not difficult at all ☐ Somewhat difficult ☐ Very difficult ☐ Extremely difficult

TOTAL SCORE _____

Personal Inventory for Depression and SAD (PIDS)

Reference: **Terman M, Terman JS, Williams JBW. Seasonal affective disorder and its treatments. J Prac Psychiatry Behav Health 1998; 5:287–303**

Rating Self-report

Administration time 15 minutes

Main purpose To screen for depression, seasonality in depressive symptoms and atypical neurovegetative symptoms.

Population Adults and adolescents

Commentary

Winter depression is a common sub-type of major depressive disorder that appears to be underdiagnosed in primary care settings. The PIDS is a 39-item self-report questionnaire developed to screen for depression and assess whether there is a seasonal component to any depressive symptoms experienced. Section 1 of the PIDS contains 11 items (adapted from the Primary Care Evaluations of Mental Disorders, page 145) that probe in a yes/no format for the presence of depressive symptoms during the previous year. Section 2 contains 7 items assessing severity of seasonal changes in mood and behaviour, and asks whether these changes represent a problem for the individual (AutoPIDS version only). Section 3 contains 12 items addressing the temporal pattern of the seasonal changes (Sections 2 and 3 adapted from the Seasonal Pattern Assessment Questionnaire, page 51). Section 4 contains 9 items probing for the presence of atypical depressive symptoms.

Scoring

Section 1: Items are scored on a yes/no format, ≥5 positive responses may indicate MDD if item 4 or 5 is endorsed. Section 2: Items are scored on a 0–4 scale, score range 0–24, with higher scores indicating greater seasonality (0–6, low seasonality; 7–11, moderate seasonality; ≥12, high seasonality). Section 3: Patients with winter depression should select the autumn/winter months in column A, summer months in Column B. Section 4: Probe for atypical symptoms (not diagnostic).

Versions

A computer administered version with on-line scoring and individualized feedback is available at www.cet.org.

Additional references

Terman M, Williams JBW. Assessment instruments. In: Seasonal Affective Disorder: Practice and Research. Partonen T, Magnússon A, Eds. Oxford, Oxford University Press 2001; 143–9.

Terman M, White T, Williams JBW. Automated Personal Inventory for Depression and SAD (AutoPIDS). Center for Environmental Therapeutics, www.cet.org.

Address for correspondence

Dr. Michael Terman
Department of Psychiatry, Columbia University
1051 Riverside Drive, Unit 50
New York, NY 10032, USA
email: mt12@columbia.edu
Website: www.cet.org.

The PIDS is available with on-line scoring on the Center for Environmental Therapeutics Website (www.cet.org). It is also available as part of the clinicians' and self-assessment forms as part of the Clinical Assessment Instruments package published and distributed by CET.

Personal Inventory for Depression and SAD (PIDS)

Name_____   Date _____

This questionnaire is designed to help determine the scope and timing of certain problems that many people have, and to help your clinician advise you about possible treatments, depending on your responses. This is not a method for self-diagnosis, but it does provide a quick way to identify personal problem areas that may deserve special attention. Circle your responses to the right of each question. Circle a "yes" or "no" response only if you are quite sure about it; if you are unsure, circle a question mark if it is given as an alternative. All information you provide is confidential.

PART 1. SOME QUESTIONS ABOUT DEPRESSION.

In the last year, have you had any single period of time – <u>lasting at least two weeks</u> – in which any of the following problems was present nearly every day? (Of course, you may also have had several such periods.)

Were there two weeks or more . . .

• when you had trouble falling asleep or staying asleep, or sleeping too much?	YES	NO	?
• when you were feeling tired or had little energy?	YES	NO	?
• when you experienced poor appetite or overeating? Or significant weight gain or loss, although you were not dieting?	YES	NO	?
• when you found little interest or little pleasure in doing things?	YES	NO	?
• when you were feeling down, depressed, or hopeless?	YES	NO	?
• when you were feeling bad about yourself – or that you were a failure – or that you were letting yourself or your family down?	YES	NO	?
• when you had trouble concentrating on things, like reading the newspaper or watching television?	YES	NO	?
• when you were so fidgety or restless that you were moving around a lot more than usual? Or the opposite – moving or speaking so slowly that other people could have noticed?	YES	NO	?
• when you found yourself thinking a lot about death or that you would be better off dead, or even of hurting yourself?	YES	NO	?

> Leave this box blank.
> y____   n____   ?____

PART 2. HOW 'SEASONAL' A PERSON ARE YOU?

Circle <u>one</u> number on each line to indicate how much each of the following behaviors or feelings <u>changes with the seasons</u>.
(For instance, you may find you sleep different hours in the winter than in the summer. *(0 = no change, 1 = slight change, 2 = moderate change, 3 = marked change, 4 = extreme change.)*

Change in your total sleep length (including nighttime sleep and naps)	0	1	2	3	4
Change in your level of social activity (including friends, family and co-workers)	0	1	2	3	4
Change in your general mood, or overall feeling of well-being	0	1	2	3	4
Change in your weight	0	1	2	3	4
Change in your appetite (both food cravings and the amount you eat)	0	1	2	3	4
Change in your energy level	0	1	2	3	4

> Leave this box blank.
> tot____

continued overleaf

PART 3. WHICH MONTHS STAND OUT AS 'EXTREME' FOR YOU?

For each of the following behaviors or feelings, draw a circle around all applicable months. If no particular month stands out for any item, circle "none". You should circle a month only if you recollect a distinct change in comparison to other months, occurring for several years. You may circle several months for each item.

COLUMN A

I tend to feel worst in — Jan Feb Mar Apr May Jun Jul Aug Sep Oct Nov Dec none

I tend to eat most in — Jan Feb Mar Apr May Jun Jul Aug Sep Oct Nov Dec none

I tend to gain most weight in — Jan Feb Mar Apr May Jun Jul Aug Sep Oct Nov Dec none

I tend to sleep most in — Jan Feb Mar Apr May Jun Jul Aug Sep Oct Nov Dec none

I tend to have the least energy in — Jan Feb Mar Apr May Jun Jul Aug Sep Oct Nov Dec none

I tend to have the lowest level of social activity in — Jan Feb Mar Apr May Jun Jul Aug Sep Oct Nov Dec none

COLUMN B

I tend to feel best in — Jan Feb Mar Apr May Jun Jul Aug Sep Oct Nov Dec none

I tend to eat least in — Jan Feb Mar Apr May Jun Jul Aug Sep Oct Nov Dec none

I tend to lose most weight in — Jan Feb Mar Apr May Jun Jul Aug Sep Oct Nov Dec none

I tend to sleep least in — Jan Feb Mar Apr May Jun Jul Aug Sep Oct Nov Dec none

I tend to have the most energy in — Jan Feb Mar Apr May Jun Jul Aug Sep Oct Nov Dec none

I tend to have the highest level of social activity in — Jan Feb Mar Apr May Jun Jul Aug Sep Oct Nov Dec none

Leave this box blank.												
	J	F	M	A	M	J	J	A	S	O	N	D	none
A	—	—	—	—	—	—	—	—	—	—	—	—	—
B	—	—	—	—	—	—	—	—	—	—	—	—	—

PART 4. MORE ABOUT POSSIBLE WINTER SYMPTOMS . . .

In comparison to other times of the year, during the winter months, which – if any – of the following symptoms tend to be present?

I tend to sleep longer hours (napping included).	YES	NO	?
I tend to have trouble waking up in the morning.	YES	NO	?
I tend to have low daytime energy, feeling tired most of the time.	YES	NO	?
I tend to feel worse, overall, in the late evening than in the morning.	YES	NO	?
I tend to have a distinct temporary slump in mood or energy in the afternoon.	YES	NO	?
I tend to crave more sweets and starches.	YES	NO	?
I tend to eat more sweets and starches, whether or not I crave them.	YES	NO	?
I tend to crave sweets, but mostly in the afternoon and evening.	YES	NO	?
I tend to gain more weight than in the summer.	YES	NO	?

Leave this box blank.
y___ n___ ?___

Michael Terman, Ph.D., and Janet B.W. Williams, D.S.W.
New York State Psychiatric Institute and
Department of Psychiatry Columbia University

SCORING INSTRUCTIONS

Tabulate ratings in the boxed space below each set of questions.
   Part 1: Total the number, separately, of "yes", "no", and "?" responses.
   Part 2: Total the circled ratings for the six questions. {SPAQ Global Seasonality Score; see Notes, below.)
   Part 3: For Column A and B, separately, total the number of times each month (or "none") was circled.
   Part 4: Total the number, separately, of "yes", "no", and "?" responses.

INTERPRETATION GUIDE

The following text is reprinted from the self-assessment version of this instrument (PIDS-SA), and is thus written in a way that directly advises the respondent. For additional information about diagnosis and treatment of SAD and related syndromes, see: Terman M, Terman JS, Williams JBW. Seasonal affective disorder and its treatments. *Journal of Practical Psychiatry and Behavioral Health* 1998;5:387–403. (Reprints available by request on letterhead to: Clinical Chronobiology Program, New York State Psychiatric Institute, 1051 Riverside Drive, Unit 50, New York, NY 10032.) The instrument is also available with online automated scoring with personalized feedback at www.cet.org.

   PART 1. If you circled 5 or more problems, it is possible that you have had a major depressive disorder for which you should consider seeking help. Even if you circled only one or two problems you may want to consult with a psychiatrist, psychologist, social worker or other mental health professional if the problems worry you or interfere with your daily activities. You may have experienced some of these problems for less than two weeks – if so, your problem is probably not a classic 'major' depressive disorder, but still may be serious enough to merit consultation with a therapist and possibly treatment. To determine whether the problem might be seasonal, consider Parts 2 and 3 below.

   PART 2. If your total score on Part 2 is less than 6, you fall within the 'nonseasonal' range. You probably do not have seasonal affective disorder (SAD). It is still possible, however, that you have experienced a chronic or intermittent depression that merits clinical attention. If your score falls between 7 and 11, you may have a mild version of SAD for which seasonal changes are noticeable – and possibly even quite bothersome – but are probably not overwhelmingly difficult. If your score is 12 or more, SAD that is clinically significant is increasingly likely. But you still need to consider which months pose most problems, as shown in Part 3.

   PART 3. People with fall or winter depression tend to score 4 or more per month in a series of 3–5 months beginning anywhere from September to January, as would be noted in Column A. For months outside that grouping the score tends to be zero, or nearly zero. In Column B, the same people will usually score 4 or more points per month over a series of 3-5 months beginning anywhere from March to June.

   Some people show a different pattern, with scores split between Columns A and B during both winter and summer months. For example, they may feel worst and socialize least during the summer, especially July and August; during the same time period, they may eat least, lose most weight, and sleep least. In winter, they may feel best and socialize most, yet still tend to eat most, gain most weight, and sleep most. Such people may experience seasonal depression of the summer type, and treatment recommendations may well differ from those for winter depression.

   Some people show relatively high scores in the fall and winter months in Column A (winter depression), but there is still a remaining scatter of good and bad months throughout the year. Such a pattern may indicate a 'winter worsening' of symptoms, rather than clear-cut SAD. Recommendations for winter treatment might be similar to those for winter-SAD, although there may be a need for multiple treatment approaches.

   Some people experience depression in the winter as well as in the summer, but they feel fine in the spring and the fall. Their summer depression is usually not accompanied by oversleeping and overeating, in contrast with the winter. This is a special case of SAD, for which different treatments might be appropriate in the opposite seasons. Even people who experience only winter depression sometimes feel summertime slumps in mood and energy when the weather is rainy or dark for several days. They often find relief by brief use of their winter treatment during these periods.

   PART 4. If you reported any of these tendencies, you have experienced winter symptoms that may respond to light therapy and various medications, regardless of whether or not you have depressed mood. The higher your score in Part 4, the more likely you are to have 'classic' winter-SAD. It is possible, however, to be depressed in winter without these symptoms – or even with opposite symptoms such as reduced sleep and appetite – if so, a therapist might recommend a different treatment from that for 'classic' SAD.

NOTES – Part 1 was adapted from the *Prime-MD Clinician Evaluation Guide (CEG)*, developed by Robert L. Spitzer, M.D., and Janet B.W. Williams, D.S.W., New York State Psychiatric Institute and Department of Psychiatry, Columbia University. Parts 2 and 3 were adapted from the *Seasonal Pattern Assessment Questionnaire (SPAQ)* developed by Norman E. Rosenthal, M.D., Gary J. Bradt, and Thomas A. Wehr, M.D., National Institute of Mental Health. Preparation of the *PIDS* was sponsored in part by Grant MH42930 from the National Institute of Mental Health. This questionnaire may not be copied for large-scale distribution without written permission of the authors. © 1993. All rights reserved. May 1993 version.

Raskin Depression Rating Scale

Reference: **Raskin A, Schulterbrandt J, Reatig N, McKeon JJ. Replication of factors of psychopathology in interview, ward behavior and self-report ratings of hospitalized depressives. J Nerv Ment Dis 1969; 148(1):87–98**

Rating Clinician-rated

Administration time 10–15 minutes

Main purpose To assess severity of depressive symptoms, with a specific focus upon verbal report, behaviour and secondary symptoms

Population Adult inpatients or outpatients

Commentary

The Raskin Depression Rating Scale (or Three-Area Severity of Depression Scale) is a brief, clinician-rated scale suitable for assessing both baseline levels of depression and change in depression severity over time. Sources of information for the rating may include patient self-report, information obtained during interview or collateral information from ward staff. The scale requires the clinician to rate the patient's verbal report of depressive symptoms, their depressed behaviour, and secondary symptoms of depression (primarily somatic). Although the Raskin scale is relatively quick and easy to administer, it lacks specificity, and is usually administered in conjunction with more specific rating scales such as the HDRS (see page 28).

Scoring

Items are rated on a 1–5 scale (1= not at all through to 5 = very much). The authors suggest that a score ≥9 represents moderate depression.

Versions

No alternative versions are available.

Additional reference

Bennie EH, Mullin JM, Martindale JJ. A double-blind multicenter trial comparing sertraline and fluoxetine in outpatients with major depression. J Clin Psychiatry 1995; 56(6):229–37.

Address for correspondence

Not applicable – the scale is in the public domain.

Raskin Depression Scale

Rate each of the following according to the degree of severity below:

    1 = Not at all
    2 = Somewhat
    3 = Moderately
    4 = Considerably
    5 = Very much

I. _____ Verbal report: Feels blue, talks of feeling helpless or worthless, complains of loss of interest, may wish to be dead, reports of crying spells.

II. _____ Behavior: Looks sad, cries easily, speaks in a sad voice, psychomotor retardation, lacking energy

III. _____ Secondary symptoms of depression: insomnia/hypersomnia, dry mouth, GI complaints, suicide attempt recently, change in appetite, cognitive problems

Reproduced from Raskin A, Schulterbrandt J, Reatig N, McKeon JJ. J Nerv Ment Dis 1969; 148(1):87–98.

Seasonal Pattern Assessment Questionnaire (SPAQ)

Reference: **Rosenthal NE, Bradt GJ, Wehr TA. Seasonal Pattern Assessment Questionnaire (SPAQ). 1984. Bethesda, MD, National Institute of Mental Health**

Rating Self-report

Administration time 5–10 minutes

Main purpose To screen for winter depression

Population Adults, adolescents and children

Commentary

The SPAQ is a brief self-report questionnaire that retrospectively assesses the magnitude of seasonal change an individual experiences in their sleep, social activity, mood, weight, appetite and energy. The scale is simple, brief and easy to use as a screening instrument, but it is not appropriate for use in isolation as a diagnostic tool, and careful clinical evaluation is still required to confirm a diagnosis of winter depression (see the Hamilton Depression Rating Scale–Seasonal Affective Disorder Version or SIGH-SAD, page 55; Personal Inventory for Depression and SAD or PIDS, page 46).

Scoring

The most commonly used section of the SPAQ provides a 'global seasonality score' (GSS), the sum of the 6 items on question 11. The GSS has a range of 0–24, with higher scores indicating more pronounced seasonality. SPAQ screening criteria for winter depression are a GSS ≥11 AND a score of 'moderate' or greater on question 17, which assesses degree of problems associated with seasonal changes. Other sections of the SPAQ record demographics, the temporal nature of patients' seasonal changes, weight and sleep fluctuation and changes in food preferences.

Versions

The SPAQ has been translated into Chinese, German, Italian, Japanese, Spanish and several Northern European languages; a modified version for children and adolescents is also available.

Additional references

Hardin TA, Wehr TA, Brewerton T, Kasper S, Berrettini W, Rabkin J, Rosenthal NE. Evaluation of seasonality in six clinical populations and two normal populations. Psychiatr Res 1991; 25(3):75–87.

Eagles JM, Wileman SM, Cameron IM, Howie FL, Lawton K, Gray DA, Andrew JE, Naji SA. Seasonal affective disorder among primary care attenders and a community sample in Aberdeen. Br J Psychiatry 1999; 175:472–5.

Michalak EE, Wilkinson C, Dowrick C, Wilkinson G. Seasonal affective disorder: prevalence, detection and current treatment in North Wales. Br J Psychiatry 2001; 179:31–4.

Young MA, Blodgett C, Reardon A. Measuring seasonality: psychometric properties of the Seasonal Pattern Assessment Questionnaire and the Inventory for Seasonal Variation. Psychiatry Res 2003; 117(1):75–83.

Address for correspondence

Dr. Norman E. Rosenthal
Clinical Professor of Psychiatry
Georgetown University Medical School
11110 Stephalee Lane
Rockville, MD 20852-3656, USA
Telephone: 1-301-770–5647
Fax: 1-301-770-6019
Email: Nermd@aol.com
Website: www.normanrosenthal.com

Seasonal Pattern Assessment Questionnaire

1. **Name** _____   2. **Age** _____

3. **Place of birth – City/Province (State)/Country** _____

4. **Today's date** _____   _____   _____
   Month   Day   Year

5. **Current weight (in lbs.)** _____

6. **Years of education**
Less than four years of high school	1
High school only	2
1–3 years post high school	3
4 or more years post high school	4

7. **Sex** –Male   1   Female   2

8. **Marital Status –**
Single	1
Married	2
Sep./Divorced	3
Widowed	4

9. **Occupation** _____

10. **How many years have you lived in this climatic area?** _____

> The purpose of this form is to find out how your mood and behaviour change over time. Please fill in all the relevant circles. Note: **We** are interested in your experience; <u>not others</u> you may have observed.

11. **To what degree do the following change with the seasons?**

	No Change	Slight Change	Moderate Change	Marked Change	Extremely Marked Change
A. Sleep length	0	1	2	3	4
B. Social activity	0	1	2	3	4
C. Mood (overall feeling of well being)	0	1	2	3	4
D. Weight	0	1	2	3	4
E. Appetite	0	1	2	3	4
F. Energy level	0	1	2	3	4

12. **In the following questions, fill in circles for all applicable months. This may be a single month ○, a cluster of months, e.g. ○ ○ ○ , or any other grouping.**

At what time of year do you....

	Jan	Feb	Mar	Apr	May	Jun	Jul	Aug	Sep	Oct	Nov	Dec	OR	No particular month(s) stand out as extreme on a regular basis
A. Feel best	○	○	○	○	○	○	○	○	○	○	○	○		○
B. Gain most weight	○	○	○	○	○	○	○	○	○	○	○	○		○
C. Socialize most	○	○	○	○	○	○	○	○	○	○	○	○		○
D. Sleep least	○	○	○	○	○	○	○	○	○	○	○	○		○
E. Eat most	○	○	○	○	○	○	○	○	○	○	○	○	**OR**	○
F. Lose most weight	○	○	○	○	○	○	○	○	○	○	○	○		○
G. Socialize least	○	○	○	○	○	○	○	○	○	○	○	○		○
H. Feel worst	○	○	○	○	○	○	○	○	○	○	○	○		○
I. Eat least	○	○	○	○	○	○	○	○	○	○	○	○		○
J. Sleep most	○	○	○	○	○	○	○	○	○	○	○	○		○

14. **How much does your weight fluctuate during the course of the year?**

0–3 lbs	1	12–15 lbs	4
4–7 lbs	2	16–20 lbs	5
8–11 lbs	3	Over 20 lbs	6

Seasonal Pattern Assessment Questionnaire (continued)

15. Approximately how many hours of each 24-hour day do you sleep during each season? (Include naps)

Winter	0	1	2	3	4	5	6	7	8	9	10	11	12	13	14	15	16	17	18	Over18
Spring	0	1	2	3	4	5	6	7	8	9	10	11	12	13	14	15	16	17	18	Over18
Summer	0	1	2	3	4	5	6	7	8	9	10	11	12	13	14	15	16	17	18	Over18
Fall	0	1	2	3	4	5	6	7	8	9	10	11	12	13	14	15	16	17	18	Over18

16. Do you notice a change in food preference during the different seasons?

No 1   Yes 2   If yes, please specify:

17. If you experience changes with the seasons, do you feel that these are a problems for you?

No 1   Yes 2   If yes, is this problem –   mild   1
 moderate   2
 marked   3
 severe   4
 disabling   5

Thank you for completing this questionnaire.

Modified by Raymond W. Lam 1998 from Rosenthal NE, Bradt GJ, Wehr TA. 1984. Bethesda, MD, National Institute of Mental Health.

Structured Interview Guide for the Hamilton Depression Rating Scale with Atypical Depression Supplement (SIGH-ADS)

Reference: **Williams JBW, Terman M. Structured Interview Guide for the Hamilton Depression Rating Scale with Atypical Depression Supplement (SIGH-ADS). New York, New York State Psychiatric Institute, 2003**

Rating Clinician-rated

Administration time 10–20 minutes depending on symptom frequency and severity

Main purpose To assess severity of, and change in, depressive symptoms including atypical symptoms of depression.

Population Adults

Commentary

The Structured Interview Guide for the Hamilton Depression Rating Scale with Atypical Depression Supplement (SIGH-ADS) supersedes the SIGH-SAD (see page 55). Designed for general use in depression research, regardless of seasonality, the SIGH-ADS questions have greater specificity, with improved question flow and presentation. Assessment of sleep symptoms is based on time estimates rather than subjective judgements (as previously), to minimize exaggeration. The scoring of the SIGH-ADS and SIGH-SAD scales is compatible, although there is also a new recommendation that 4 of the original 29 items not be included in the core depression scale total. Additional exploratory items include Difficulty Awakening and Temperature Discomfort. For each item, the boldfaced stem questions are to be read verbatim to the patient. Unbolded questions are used for further probing if needed, and the rater may elaborate on these as appropriate in individual cases.

Scoring

Total scores are separately derived for 17-item Hamilton Scale items, 8-item Atypical Scale items and the 25-item SIGH-ADS total.

Versions

Author-approved, back-translated versions are being prepared in several languages. A German translation is available (info@cet.org). The self-rating version of the SIGH-SAD, the SIGH-SAD-SR (also available in German), can be used as a reliability check on SIGH-ADS interviewer ratings; items with 2 or more points discrepancy are referred back to the rater for clarification and possible re-scoring. The interviewer's decision is final. The SIGH-SAD-SR, with demonstrated reliability gauged against the interview version, has also been used independently in outpatient studies.

Additional reference

Williams JB. A structured interview guide for the Hamilton Depression Rating Scale. Arch Gen Psychiatry 1988; 45(8):742–7.

Terman M, Williams JBW, Terman JS. Light therapy for winter depression: a clinician's guide. In: Innovations in Clinical Practice, vol. 10, Keller PA, Heyman SR, Eds. Sarasota, FL: Professional Resource Exchange. 1991, pp 179–221.

Terman M, Terman JS, Ross DC. A controlled trial of timed bright light and negative air ionization for treatment of winter depression. Arch Gen Psychiatry 1998; 55:875–82.

Terman M, Williams JBW. Assessment instruments. In: Seasonal Affective Disorder: Practice and Research. Partonen T, Magnusson A, Eds. Oxford: Oxford University Press. 2001, pp 143–9.

Address for correspondence

Dr. Michael Terman
Department of Psychiatry, Columbia University
1051 Riverside Drive, Unit 50
New York, NY 10032, USA
Telephone: 1-212-543-5712
email: mtl2@columbia.edu

The SIGH-SAD is part of the Clinical Assessment Instruments Package published and distributed by the Center for Environmental Therapeutics (www.cet.org).

Structured Interview Guide for the Hamilton Depression Rating Scale – Seasonal Affective Disorder version (SIGH-SAD)

Reference: **Williams JBW, Link MJ, Rosenthal NE, Terman M. Structured Interview Guide for the Hamilton Depression Rating Scale – Seasonal Affective Disorder version (SIGH-SAD). New York: New York State Psychiatric Institute, 2002**

Rating Clinician-rated

Administration time 10–20 minutes depending on symptom frequency and severity

Main purpose To assess severity of, and change in, depressive symptoms including atypical symptoms of depression

Population Adults

Commentary

A limitation of the HDRS or Ham-D is that atypical symptoms of depression (e.g., hypersomnia, hyperphagia) are not assessed. Originally developed for research in seasonal affective disorder, this version adds 8 items to the 21-item HDRS version (HDRS21) for use when assessment of atypical symptoms is needed. All 29 items have been used to give a total score of severity although the 8-item atypical addendum is sometimes analysed separately from the HDRS21. Other studies generate a severity score using 24 items (the HDRS17 score plus the 7 corresponding items on the 8-item atypical addendum). The recently developed SIGH-ADS (Atypical Depression Supplement – see page 54) supersedes the SIGH-SAD.

Scoring

Total scores are seperately derived for 17- or 21-item Hamilton Scale items, 7- or 8-item Atypical Scale items and the 24- or 29-item SIGH-SAD total.

Versions

A self-rating version of the Structured Interview Guide for the Hamilton Depression Rating Scale – Seasonal Affective Disorder Version (SIGH-SAD-SR) has been developed. The SIGH-SAD-SR can be used as a reliability check on SIGH-SAD interviewer ratings; items with 2 or more points discrepancy are referred back to the rater for clarification and possible re-scoring. The interviewer's decision is final. The SIGH-SAD-SR, with demonstrated reliability gauged against the interview version, has also been used independently in outpatient studies.

Additional references

Williams JB. A structured interview guide for the Hamilton Depression Rating Scale. Arch Gen Psychiatry 1988; 45(8):742–7.

Terman M, Williams JBW, Terman JS. Light therapy for winter depression: a clinician's guide. In: Innovations in Clinical Practice, vol. 10, Keller PA, Heyman SR, Eds. Sarasota, FL: Professional Resource Exchange. 1991, pp 179–221.

Terman M, Terman JS, Ross DC. A controlled trial of timed bright light and negative air ionization for treatment of winter depression. Arch Gen Psychiatry 1998; 55:875–82.

Eastman CI, Young MA, Fogg LF, Liu L, Meaden PM. Bright light treatment of winter depression: a placebo-controlled trial. Arch Gen Psychiatry 1998; 55:883–9.

Terman M, Williams JBW. Assessment instruments. In: Seasonal Affective Disorder: Practice and Research. Partonen T, Magnusson A, Eds. Oxford: Oxford University Press. 2001, pp 143–9.

Address for correspondence

Dr. Michael Terman
Department of Psychiatry, Columbia University
1051 Riverside Drive, Unit 50
New York, NY 10032, USA
Telephone: 1-212-543-5712
email: mtl2@columbia.edu

The SIGH-SAD is part of the Clinical Assessment Instruments Package published and distributed by the Center for Environmental Therapeutics (www.cet.org).

Suicide Probability Scale (SPS)

Reference: **Cull JG, Gill WS. Suicide Probability Scale (SPS) Manual. 1988. Los Angeles, CA, Western Psychological Services**

Rating Self-report

Administration time 5–10 minutes

Main purpose To assess suicide risk

Population Adults and adolescents

Commentary

The SPS is a 36-item self-report scale developed to assess suicide risk in adults and adolescents aged over 13 years. The instrument has shown moderate ability to predict future suicide attempts in adolescents in a group home setting, but its power to predict future suicide attempts in adults with mood disorders is unclear. The SPS should be used in the context of a comprehensive clinical evaluation of suicide risk.

Scoring

Items are scored on a 4-point scale, and the instrument generates 3 summary scores - a total weighted score, a normalized score, a Suicide Probability Score, and four subscales (hopelessness, suicide ideation, negative self-evaluation, and hostility). The manual provides norms for the general population, psychiatric patients, and lethal suicide attempters.

Versions

Authorized research translations of the SPS have been conducted in Malayan, Spanish, Swedish, and Turkish (though copies of the resulting translations have not been filed with WPS by the researchers). No commercial editions of the SPS are available in languages other than English.

Additional references

Cappelli M, Clulow MK, Goodman JT, Davidson SI, Feder SH, Baron P, Manion IG, McGrath PJ. Identifying depressed and suicidal adolescents in a teen health clinic. J Adolesc Health 1995; 16(1):64–70.

Larzelere RE, Smith GL, Batenhorst LM, Kelly DB. Predictive validity of the suicide probability scale among adolescents in group home treatment. J Am Acad Child Adolesc Psychiatry 1996; 35(2):166–72.

Address for correspondence

Western Psychological Services
12031 Wilshire Blvd.
Los Angeles, CA 90025-1251, USA
Telephone: 1-310-478-2061
Website: http://www.wpspublish.com
Email: custsvc@wpspublish.com

Suicide Probability Scale (SPS) – sample items

- I feel the world is not worth continuing to live in
- I feel it would be less painful to die than to keep living the way things are

Young Mania Rating Scale (YMRS)

Reference: Young RC, Biggs JT, Ziegler VE, Meyer DA. **A rating scale for mania: reliability, validity and sensitivity. Br J Psychiatry 1978; 133:429–35**

Rating Clinician-rated

Administration time 10–20 minutes

Main purpose To assess severity of manic symptoms

Population Adults and adolescents with mania

Commentary

The YMRS is an 11-item clinician-rated scale designed to assess severity of manic symptoms. The gold standard of mania rating scales, the instrument is widely used in both clinical and research settings. Information for assigning scores is gained from the patient's subjective reported symptoms over the previous 48 hours and from clinical observation during the interview. The scale is appropriate both for assessing baseline severity of manic symptoms, and response to treatment in patients with bipolar disorder type I and II. However, the YMRS does not assess concomitant depressive symptoms and should be administered in conjunction with a depression rating scale such as the HDRS (see page 28) or the MADRS (see page 39) in patients with concomitant symptoms of depression or those experiencing a mixed episode.

Scoring

Four of the YMRS items are rated on a 0–8 scale, with the remaining 5 items being rated on a 0–4 scale. Clear anchor-points are provided to help the clinician determine severity. A score of ≤12 indicates remission of symptoms.

Versions

A parent version of the YMRS has been produced; the scale has been translated into other languages including Spanish and Turkish, but the Royal College of Psychiatrists does not hold a record of currently available translations.

Additional references

Gracious BL, Youngstrom EA, Findling RL, Calabrese JR. Discriminative validity of a parent version of the Young Mania Rating Scale. J Am Acad Child Adolesc Psychiatry 2002; 41(11):1350–9.

Colom F, Vieta E, Martinez-Aran A, Reinares M, Goikolea JM, Benabarre A, Torrent C, Comes M, Corbella B, Parramon G, Corominas J. A randomized trial on the efficacy of group psychoeducation in the prophylaxis of recurrences in bipolar patients whose disease is in remission. Arch Gen Psychiatry 2003; 60(4):402–7.

Tohen M, Goldberg JF, Gonzalez-Pinto Arrillaga AM, Azorin JM, Vieta E, Hardy-Bayle MC, Lawson WB, Emsley RA, Zhang F, Baker RW, Risser RC, Namjoshi MA, Evans AR, Breier A. A 12-week, double-blind comparison of olanzapine vs haloperidol in the treatment of acute mania. Arch Gen Psychiatry 2003; 60(12):1218–26.

Address for correspondence

The Royal College of Psychiatrists
The British Journal of Psychiatry
17 Belgrave Square, London SW1X 8PG, UK
Telephone: +44 (20) 7235 2351
Email: publications@rcpsych.ac.uk

Young Mania Rating Scale (YMRS)

Enter the appropriate score which best characterizes the subject for each item.

Item	Explanation
1. Elevated mood	0 absent 1 mildly or possibly increased on questioning 2 definite subjective elevation: optimistic, self-confident; cheerful; appropriate to content 3 elevated, inappropriate to content; humorous 4 euphoric, inappropriate laughter singing
2. Increased motor activity-energy	0 absent 1 subjectively increased 2 animated; gestures increased 3 excessive energy; hyperactive at times; restless (can be calmed) 4 motor excitement; continues hyperactivity (cannot be calmed)
3. Sexual interest	0 normal; not increased 1 mildly or possibly increased 2 definite subjective increase on questioning 3 spontaneous sexual content; elaborates on sexual matters; hypersexual by self-report 4 overt sexual acts (toward subjects, staff, or interviewer)
4. Sleep	0 reports no decrease in sleep 1 sleeping less than normal amount by up to one hour 2 sleeping less than normal by more than one hour 3 reports decreased need for sleep 4 denies need for sleep
5. Irritability	0 absent 2 subjectively increased 4 irritable at times during interview; recent episodes of anger or annoyance on ward 6 frequently irritable during interview; short, curt throughout 8 hostile, uncooperative; interview impossible
6. Speech (rate and amount)	0 no increase 2 feels talkative 4 increased rate or amount at times, verbose at times 6 push; consistently increased rate and amount; difficult to interpret 8 pressured; uninterruptible; continuous speech
7. Language-thought disorder	0 absent 1 circumstantial; mild distractibility; quick thoughts 2 distractible; loses goal of thought; changes topics frequently; racing thoughts 3 flight of ideas; tangentiality; difficult to follow; rhyming; echolalia 4 incoherent; communication impossible
8. Content	0 normal 2 questionable plans, new interests 4 special project(s); hyperreligious 6 grandiose or paranoid ideas; ideas of reference 8 delusions; hallucinations
9. Disruptive-aggressive behaviour	0 absent, cooperative 2 sarcastic; loud at times, guarded 4 demanding; threats on ward 6 threatens interviewer shouting; interview difficult 8 assaultive; destructive; interview impossible
10. Appearance	0 appropriate dress and grooming 1 minimally unkempt 2 poorly groomed; moderately disheveled; overdressed 3 disheveled; partly clothed; garish make-up 4 completely unkempt; decorated; bizarre garb
11. Insight	0 present; admits illness; agrees with need for treatment 1 possibly ill 2 admits behaviour change, but denies illness 3 admits possible change in behaviour, but denies illness 4 denies any behaviour change

Reproduced from Young RC, Biggs JT, Ziegler VE, Meyer DA. Br J Psychiatry 1978; 133:429–35 with permission from the Royal College of Psychiatrists.

Zung Self-Rating Depression Scale (Zung SDS)

Reference: **Zung WW. A self-rating depression scale. Arch Gen Psychiatry 1965; 12:63–70**

Rating Self-report (Zung SDS) or clinician-rated (Zung DSI)

Administration time 5 minutes

Main purpose To assess depressive symptomatology

Population Adults and adolescents

Commentary

The Zung SDS is a 20-item self-report measure of depressive symptoms over the past week in adults. A clinician-rated version, the Depression Status Inventory (DSI) is also available, and contains the same 20 items. Advantages of the Zung SDS include its ease of administration and brevity. It shows good psychometric properties as a screening tool for depression, and has been used to assess outcome in response to treatment in a wide range of research studies. Disadvantages include its lack of assessment of atypical symptoms of depression.

Scoring

Half of the items in the Zung SDS are worded positively, half negatively, with positive items being scored on a 1–4 scale, negative items on a 4–1 scale according to the amount of time symptoms have been experienced during the past week. The scale has a score range of 20–80, with higher scores indicating greater depression severity. An index score can be derived by dividing the raw score by the maximum possible score. Suggested severity ranges are: <50, normal range; 50–59, mild depression; 60–69, moderate to marked depression; >70, severe depression.

Versions

The scale has been translated into Dutch, Finnish, German, Greek and Spanish, amongst other languages (see Naughton and Wiklund, 1993 for review). A modified version that assesses depressive symptoms over the past week and incorporates slight changes to the instrument's rating scale is available in the Early Clinical Drug Evaluation Manual (Guy, 1976).

Additional references

Zung WW. The Depression Status Inventory: an adjunct to the Self-Rating Depression Scale. J Clin Psychol 1972; 28(4):539–43.

Guy W, editor. ECDEU Assessment Manual for Psychopharmacology. 1976. Rockville, MD, U.S. Department of Health, Education, and Welfare.

Zung WW. The role of rating scales in the identification and management of the depressed patient in the primary care setting. J Clin Psychiatry 1990; 51 Suppl:72–6.

Naughton MJ, Wiklund I. A critical review of dimension-specific measures of health-related quality of life in cross-cultural research. Qual Life Res 1993; 2(6):397–432.

Address for correspondence

None available

ZUNG SDS (ECDEU version)

INSTRUCTIONS

Listed below are 20 statements. Please read each one carefully and decide how much of the statement describes how you have been feeling during the past week. Decide whether the statement applies to you for NONE OR A LITTLE OF THE TIME, SOME OF THE TIME, A GOOD PART OF THE TIME, OR MOST OR ALL OF THE TIME. Mark the appropriate column for each statement.

Statement	None or a little of the time	Some of the time	A good part of the time	Most or all of the time
1. I feel downhearted and blue	_____	_____	_____	_____
2. Morning is when I feel the best	_____	_____	_____	_____
3. I have crying spells or feel like it	_____	_____	_____	_____
4. I have trouble sleeping at night	_____	_____	_____	_____
5. I eat as much as I used to	_____	_____	_____	_____
6. I still enjoy sex	_____	_____	_____	_____
7. I notice that I am losing weight	_____	_____	_____	_____
8. I have trouble with constipation	_____	_____	_____	_____
9. My heart beats faster than usual	_____	_____	_____	_____
10. I get tired for no reason	_____	_____	_____	_____
11. My mind is as clear as it used to be	_____	_____	_____	_____
12. I find it easy to do the things I used to do	_____	_____	_____	_____
13. I am restless and can't keep still	_____	_____	_____	_____
14. I feel hopeful about the future	_____	_____	_____	_____
15. I am more irritable than usual	_____	_____	_____	_____
16. I find it easy to make decisions	_____	_____	_____	_____
17. I feel that I am useful and needed	_____	_____	_____	_____
18. My life is pretty full	_____	_____	_____	_____
19. I feel that others would be better off if I were dead	_____	_____	_____	_____
20. I still enjoy the things I used to do	_____	_____	_____	_____

Reproduced from Zung WW. Arch Gen Psychiatry 1965; 12:63–70.

Chapter 3

Anxiety

Fearful, scared, unnerved, nervous, restless, agitated, edgy, panicky, tense, shaky, abuzz, terrified, hypervigilant, worried, petrified, afraid, timid, shy, apprehensive, concerned, fretful, twitchy, impatient, disturbed, uptight, shocked, stressed, distraught, fidgety, distressed, disconcerted, confused, perturbed, jumpy, tremulous, overwrought, troubled, vexed, bothered, alarmed, upset, horrified, uneasy, mithered.

There are so many words to describe anxiety. Fear is obviously a universal human experience that, from an evolutionary perspective, must serve a highly adaptive purpose to be so conserved. Indeed, anxiety serves as a signal in response to stressful situations to activate stress hormones via the hypothalamic-pituitary-adrenal axis and prepare for the fight-versus-flight response. Anxiety can focus attention and concentration to improve performance, but excessive and/or prolonged anxiety can lead to changes in thinking and behaviour, overactive stress hormone release, and degradation in functioning.

Anxiety disorders are common in the general population, and they are also frequently comorbid with major depression. The central feature of these disorders is, by definition, anxiety – pervasive feelings of nervousness or tension. Individual anxiety disorders are categorized by the specific nature of the anxiety or the stimulus that produces anxiety (Table 3.1).

Panic disorder and agoraphobia

Panic disorder is characterized by panic attacks, in which there is sudden onset of extreme anxiety associated with symptoms of autonomic hyperactivity, including tachycardia or palpitations, tremulousness, shortness of breath, dizziness, vertigo, and sweating (Table 3.2). These symptoms are severe enough that patients often feel like they are having a heart attack, or that they are dying or that something terrible is about to happen, leading to frequent emergency room visits. The episodes peak quickly but also resolve quickly, with a typical duration of 20 minutes or less, although resolution of all symptoms may take longer.

With increasing frequency of panic attacks, patients begin to be fearful of future attacks, termed anticipatory anxiety. The anticipatory anxiety leads to avoidance behaviour in which situations that are believed to trigger panic attacks are avoided, or where people feel they cannot get help quickly. Hence, they increasingly avoid being alone and being in crowded places where they believe that others will think they are crazy. This can lead to agoraphobia and house-bound behaviour (Table 3.3). Agoraphobia without a history of panic attacks is much less frequently seen.

Table 3.1 Key features of anxiety disorders

Anxiety disorder	Key features
• Generalized anxiety disorder	• Anxiety and worry without a significant identified source
• Panic disorder	• Acute panic attacks
	• Anticipatory anxiety
• Obsessive-compulsive disorder	• Repetitive thoughts and actions or rituals
• Social anxiety disorder	• Anxiety in social situations with a fear of negative appraisal
• Post traumatic stress disorder	• Anxiety related to a previous life-threatening event

---

Table 3.2 Summary of DSM-IV-TR symptom criteria for panic attacks

- A discrete period of intense fear or discomfort, in which four (or more) of the following symptoms developed abruptly and reached a peak within 10 minutes.
  1. palpitations, pounding heart, or rapid heart rate
  2. sweating
  3. trembling or shaking
  4. sensations of shortness of breath or smothering
  5. feeling of choking
  6. chest pain or discomfort
  7. nausea or abdominal distress
  8. feeling dizzy, unsteady, lightheaded, or faint
  9. derealization (feelings of unreality) or depersonalization (being detached from oneself)
  10. fear of losing control or going crazy
  11. fear of dying
  12. paresthesias (numbness or tingling sensations)
  13. chills or hot flushes

Generalized anxiety disorder

Generalized anxiety disorder (GAD) is the most common anxiety disorder seen in primary care and it is frequently comorbid with depression. In this condition, there are non-specific symptoms of inner tension together with uncontrollable worrying. Compared to panic disorder, GAD has fewer somatic symptoms of autonomic hyperactivity (Table 3.4). These anxiety symptoms are usually present throughout the day. If the symptoms worsen, they do so in a 'slow wave' rather than a 'sudden spike' of symptoms.

Social phobia (social anxiety disorder)

Other anxiety disorders include specific phobias (fear of flying, crossing bridges, blood, insects, are common), social anxiety disorder (also known as social phobia) and post traumatic stress disorder. Social anxiety disorder is characterized by excessive anxiety in social situations and can be very debilitating (Table 3.5). Fear in social phobia

can be confined to a specific situation (e.g., public speaking, public washrooms, writing in front of others) or can be generalized (experienced in most social situations).

Obsessive–compulsive disorder

Obsessive–compulsive disorder (OCD) includes the presence of obsessions, which are senseless repetitive and intrusive thoughts, and/or compulsions, which are repetitive acts that serve to reduce anxiety and ward off obsessions (Table 3.6). Common obsessions include fear of

Table 3.7 Summary of DSM-IV-TR symptom criteria for post traumatic stress disorder

- The person has been exposed to a traumatic event in which both of the following were present:
  1 the person experienced or witnessed an event that involved actual or threatened death or serious injury (including physical and sexual abuse)
  2 the person's response involved intense fear, helplessness, or horror.

- The traumatic event is persistently reexperienced in one (or more) of the following ways:
  1 recurrent and intrusive distressing recollections of the event, including images, thoughts, or perceptions.
  2 recurrent distressing dreams of the event.
  3 acting or feeling as if the traumatic event were recurring (includes a sense of reliving the experience, illusions, hallucinations, and dissociative flashback episodes).
  4 Intense psychological distress at exposure to internal or external cues that symbolize or resemble an aspect of the traumatic event
  5 Physiological reactivity on exposure to internal or external cues that symbolize or resemble an aspect of the traumatic event

- Persistent avoidance of stimuli associated with the trauma and numbing of general responsiveness (not present before the trauma), as indicated by three (or more) of the following:
  1 efforts to avoid thoughts, feelings, or conversations associated with the trauma
  2 efforts to avoid activities, places, or people that arouse recollections of the trauma
  3 inability to recall an important aspect of the trauma
  4 markedly diminished interest or participation in significant activities
  5 feeling of detachment or estrangement from others
  6 restricted range of affect (e.g., unable to have loving feelings)
  7 sense of a foreshortened future (e.g., does not expect to have a career, marriage, children, or a normal life span)

- Persistent symptoms of increased arousal (not present before the trauma), as indicated by two (or more) of the following:
  1 difficulty falling or staying asleep
  2 irritability or outbursts of anger
  3 difficulty concentrating
  4 hypervigilance
  5 exaggerated startle response

germs, harming others, violent images and sexual images. Common compulsions relate to handwashing, checking rituals, counting, and the need for order. These rituals can become extremely intricate. Patients initially resist the obsessions and compulsions, although later in the course of OCD there may be less resistance. They also usually have insight as to the senselessness of their obsessions, although again later in the illness course they may lose insight. Obsessions may then become delusion-like, with a shift into obsessive compulsive disorder with overvalued ideation (OCV). Patients with OCD are at times very reluctant to reveal or discuss their symptoms because of their seemingly bizarre nature.

Post traumatic stress disorder

Post traumatic stress disorder (PTSD) is comprised of anxiety related to a significant, life-threatening stressor such as a motor vehicle accident, violent assault, or war. Characteristic symptoms include reliving the trauma through flashbacks or nightmares, hypervigilance to the environment, and affective blunting (Table 3.7). Other associated symptoms of PTSD include avoidance of situations or cues that recall the trauma, feelings of detachment, floating, or dissociation, and hopelessness for the future.

Adult Manifest Anxiety Scale (AMAS)

Reference: **Reynolds CR, Richmond BO, and Lowe PA. The Adult Manifest Anxiety Scale: Professional Manual. 2003. Los Angeles, CA, Western Psychological Services**

Rating Self-report

Administration time 10 minutes

Main purpose To assess the level and nature of anxiety in adults

Population Adults, college students and older adults

Commentary

The AMAS is a self-report instrument that is available in 3 versions: the AMAS-A for adults (19 to 59 years); the AMAS-E for elderly individuals (60 years and above); and the AMAS-C for college students. The 3 forms (containing between 36 and 49 items) were independently developed, and each includes some unique items and/or subscales. The AMAS-A, for example, contains several items addressing work pressures, while the AMAS-E includes items focusing on fear of aging. The AMAS-A and the AMAS-E yield 3 sub-scales: worry/oversensitivity, social concerns/stress and physiological anxiety, and worry/oversensitivity, social concerns/stress and fear of aging respectively. The AMAS-C yields 4 sub-scales: worry/oversensitivity, social concerns/stress and physiological anxiety and test anxiety. The AMAS was standardized on a nationally stratified random sample of individuals. The manual (Reynolds et al., 2003) reports several validity studies as well as factor analytic data supporting the structure of the 3 versions of the AMAS and its relationship to other measures of psychopathology. The scale offers a brief, simple method for assessing anxiety in adults across the age spectrum.

Scoring

Items are scored in a yes/no format; responses are summed to obtain total scores and sub-scale scores. All versions include a Lie Scale.

Versions

The instrument has not been translated into any other languages.

Additional references

Lowe PA and Reynolds CR. Exploratory analyses of the latent structure of anxiety among older adults. Educ Psychol Meas 2000; 60:100–16.

Lowe PA and Reynolds CR. Psychometric analyses of the AMAS-A among young and middle-aged adults. Educ Psychol Meas 2004; 64:661–81.

Address for correspondence

Western Psychological Services
12031 Wilshire Blvd.
Los Angeles, CA 90025-1251, USA
Telephone: 1-310-478-2061
Email: custsvc@wpspubish.com
Website: http://www.wpspublish.com

Adult Manifest Anxiety Scale – sample items

- I often worry about what could happen to my family.

- I feel keyed up or on edge a lot.

- Sometimes I worry about things that don't really matter.

- I am always good.

Anxiety Sensitivity Index (ASI)

Reference: **Peterson RA, Reiss S. Anxiety Sensitivity Index Revised Test Manual. 1993. Worthington, OH, IDS Publishing Corporation**

Rating Self-report

Administration time <5 minutes

Main purpose To measure anxiety sensitivity

Population Adults, adolescents, and older adults

Commentary

The ASI is a 16-item self report measure of anxiety sensitivity, or fear of anxiety-related symptoms based on beliefs about their potential harmful consequences. More than 100 peer-reviewed articles have demonstrated that high anxiety sensitivity is related to panic attacks, panic disorder, and posttraumatic stress disorder (PTSD). In evaluating anxiety conditions, it may be helpful to consider not just the amount of anxiety experienced by the patient, but also their sensitivity to anxiety; the ASI represents a rapid and psychometrically sound instrument for measuring anxiety sensitivity and response to treatment in patients with panic disorder. Although not a diagnostic measure, the ASI can be used to distinguish patients with panic disorder from patients with other anxiety disorders.

Scoring

Items are rated on a 0 (very little) to 5 (very much) scale, a total score (range 0–64) for the scale is derived by summing all items.

Versions

The ASI has been translated into over 20 languages, including Chinese, Dutch, German, Hebrew, Italian and Spanish. An 18-item child version (the Childhood Anxiety Sensitivity Index or CASI) is available, as well as several modified versions such as the 4-item Brief Panic Disorder Screen (BPDS), a 23-item version and a revised 36-item version (see page 66). A computer administered version is also available.

Additional references

Reiss S, Peterson RA, Gursky DM, McNally RJ. Anxiety sensitivity, anxiety frequency and the prediction of fearfulness. Behav Res Ther 1986; 24(1):1–8.

Apfeldorf WJ, Shear MK, Leon AC, Portera L. A brief screen for panic disorder. J Anxiety Disord 1994; 8:71–8.

Peterson RA and Plehn K. Measuring Anxiety Sensitivity. In S. Taylor (Ed.) Anxiety Sensitivity: Theory, Research and Treatment of the Fear of Anxiety. 1999. Hillsdale, NY: Lawrence Erlbaum Associates Publishers, pages 61–81.

McNally RJ. Anxiety sensitivity and panic disorder. Biol Psychiatry 2002; 52(10):938–46.

Address for correspondence

IDS Publishing Corporation
P.O. Box 389
Worthington, OH 43085, USA.
Telephone: 1-614-885-2323
Email: sales@idspublishing.com
Website: www.idspublishing.com

Anxiety Sensitivity Index–Revised 36 (ASI-R-36)

Reference: **Taylor S, Cox BJ. An expanded anxiety sensitivity index: evidence for a hierarchic structure in a clinical sample. J Anxiety Disord 1998; 12(5):463–83**

Rating Self-report

Administration time 5 minutes

Main purpose To assess anxiety sensitivity

Population Adults and adolescents

Commentary

The ASI-R-36 is a revised version of the original Anxiety Sensitivity Index (see page 65), of which 10 items were retained; the 26 new items on the ASI-R-36 were developed to more adequately assess the somatic, cognitive and social dimensions of anxiety sensitivity. The scale possesses 6 sub-scales assessing fear of: cardiovascular symptoms, respiratory symptoms, gastrointestinal symptoms, publicly observable anxiety reactions, dissociative and neurological symptoms, and fear of cognitive dyscontrol.

Scoring

Items are rated on a 5-point scale ranging from 0 (very little) to 4 (very much); a total score (range 0–144) for the scale is derived by summing all items.

Versions

The ASI-R-36 has been translated into Dutch, French, Icelandic, Spanish and Turkish.

Additional references

Stewart SH, Taylor S, Jang KL, Cox BJ, Watt MC, Fedoroff IC, Borger SC. Causal modeling of relations among learning history, anxiety sensitivity, and panic attacks. Behav Res Ther 2001; 39:443–56.

Zvolensky MJ, Arrindell WA, Taylor S, Bouvard M, Cox BJ, Stewart SH, Sandin B, Cardenas SJ, Eifert GH. Anxiety sensitivity in six countries. Behav Res Ther 2003; 41(7):841–59.

Address for correspondence

Dr. Steven Taylor
Department of Psychiatry
University of British Columbia
2255 Wesbrook Mall
Vancouver, V6T 2A1, Canada
Telephone: 1-604-822-7331
Email: taylor@interchange.ubc.ca

Please circle the number that best corresponds to how much you agree with each item. If any of the items concern something that is not part of your experience (for example, "It scares me when I feel shaky" for someone who has never trembled or felt shaky) answer on the basis of who you expect you think you might feel <u>if you had</u> such an experience. Otherwise, answer all items on the basis of your own experience. Be careful to circle only one number for each item and please answer all items.

	Very little	A little	Some	Much	Very much
1. It is important for me not to appear nervous	0	1	2	3	4
2. When I cannot keep my mind on a task, I worry that I might be going crazy	0	1	2	3	4
3. It scares me when I feel "shaky" (trembling)	0	1	2	3	4
4. It scares me when I feel faint	0	1	2	3	4
5. It scares me when my heart beats rapidly	0	1	2	3	4
6. It scares me when I am nauseous	0	1	2	3	4
7. When I notice that my heart is beating rapidly, I worry that I might have a heart attack	0	1	2	3	4
8. It scares me when I become short of breath	0	1	2	3	4
9. When my stomach is upset, I worry that I might be seriously ill	0	1	2	3	4
10. It scares me when I am unable to keep my mind on a task	0	1	2	3	4
11. When my head is pounding, I worry I could have a stroke	0	1	2	3	4
12. When I tremble in the presence of others, I fear what people might think of me	0	1	2	3	4
13. When I feel like I'm not getting enough air, I get scared that I might suffocate	0	1	2	3	4
14. When I get diarrhea, I worry that I might have something wrong with me	0	1	2	3	4
15. When my chest feels tight, I get scared that I won't be able to breathe properly	0	1	2	3	4
16. When my breathing becomes irregular, I fear that something bad will happen	0	1	2	3	4
17. It frightens me when my surroundings seem strange or unreal	0	1	2	3	4
18. Smothering sensations scare me	0	1	2	3	4
19. When I feel pain in my chest, I worry that I'm going to have a heart attack	0	1	2	3	4
20. I believe it would be awful to vomit in public	0	1	2	3	4
21. It scares me when my body feels strange or different in some way	0	1	2	3	4
22. I worry that other people will notice my anxiety	0	1	2	3	4
23. When I feel "spacey" or spaced out I worry that I may be mentally ill	0	1	2	3	4
24. It scares me when I blush in front of people	0	1	2	3	4
25. When I feel a strong pain in my stomach, I worry it could be cancer	0	1	2	3	4
26. When I have trouble swallowing, I worry that I could choke	0	1	2	3	4
27. When I notice my heart skipping a beat, I worry that there is something seriously wrong with me	0	1	2	3	4
28. It scares me when I feel tingling or prickling sensations in my hands	0	1	2	3	4
29. When I feel dizzy, I worry there is something wrong with my brain	0	1	2	3	4
30. When I begin to sweat in a social situation, I fear people will think negatively of me	0	1	2	3	4
31. When my thoughts seem to speed up, I worry that I might be going crazy	0	1	2	3	4
32. When my throat feels tight, I worry that I could choke to death	0	1	2	3	4
33. When my face feels numb, I worry that I might be having a stroke	0	1	2	3	4
34. When I have trouble thinking clearly, I worry that there is something wrong with me	0	1	2	3	4
35. I think it would be horrible for me to faint in public	0	1	2	3	4
36. When my mind goes blank, I worry there is something terribly wrong with me.	0	1	2	3	4

Reproduced from Taylor S, Cox BJ. J Anxiety Disord 1988; 12:463–83 with permission from Elsevier.

Beck Anxiety Inventory (BAI)

Reference: **Beck AT, Epstein N, Brown G, Steer RA. An inventory for measuring clinical anxiety: psychometric properties. J Consult Clin Psychol 1988; 56(6):893–7**

Rating Self-report

Administration time 5–10 minutes

Main purpose To assess symptoms of anxiety (particularly somatic)

Population Adults and adolescents

Commentary

The BAI is a widely used 21-item self-report measure designed to assess severity of anxious symptoms over the past week. Each item describes a common symptom of anxiety such as heart pounding or racing, inability to relax and dizziness. The scale was designed to discriminate depression from anxiety, and emphasizes the more somatic, panic-type symptoms of anxiety, rather than symptoms of generalized anxiety, such as worry, sleep disturbance or poor concentration. Although the BAI shows substantial correlations with measures of depression such as the Beck Depression Inventory (see page 10) and the depression sub-scale of the Symptom Checklist-90-R (see page 166), it appears to discriminate more accurately between anxiety and depression than some other anxiety measures, such as the State-Trait Anxiety Inventory (see page 109). The BAI is a reliable and widely-used screen for somatic anxiety symptoms that is sensitive to treatment response, although it is not appropriate for the assessment of generalized anxiety disorder (GAD).

Scoring

Items are scored on a 0 (not at all) to 3 (severely: I could barely stand it) scale, with a score range of 0–63. Scores of 0–7 represent minimal anxiety, 8–15, mild anxiety, 16–25, moderate anxiety and 26–63, severe anxiety.

Versions

The BAI has been translated into Chinese, Danish, Finnish, French, German and Portuguese. A computer-administered version is available.

Additional references

Beck AT, Epstein N, Brown G, Steer RA. An inventory for measuring clinical anxiety: psychometric properties. J Consult Clin Psychol 1988; 56(6):893–7.

Cox BJ, Cohen E, Direnfeld DM, Swinson RP. Does the Beck Anxiety Inventory measure anything beyond panic attack symptoms? Behav Res Ther 1996; 34(11–12):949–54.

Address for correspondence

Harcourt Assessment, Inc.
19500 Bulverde Road
San Antonio, TX 78259, USA
Telephone: 1-800–2111-8378
Website: www.HarcourtAssessment.com

Brief Social Phobia Scale (BSPS)

Reference: **Davidson JR, Potts NL, Richichi EA, Ford SM, Krishnan KR, Smith RD, Wilson W. The Brief Social Phobia Scale. J Clin Psychiatry 1991; 52 Suppl:48–51**

Rating Clinician-rated

Administration time 5–15 minutes

Main purpose To assess fear, avoidance and physiological arousal related to social phobia

Population Adults

Commentary

The BPRS is an 11-item observer-rated scale measure of social phobia symptom severity over the previous week. The scale consists of 7 items measuring specific phobic situations from the perspective of both fear and avoidance and 4 further items evaluating physiological symptoms experienced while exposed to or thinking about the phobic situation. The scale developers recommend that the BPRS be administered after a clinical interview; if no exposure to a particular phobic situation has occurred in the previous week, the patient should be asked to imagine how he or she would feel if exposed to that situation now. The BPRS represents a brief and efficient scale for social phobia. It has been used as an outcome measure in a variety of pharmaceutical trials and provides a shorter alternative to the Liebowitz Social Anxiety Scale (see page 84) for evaluating social phobia. However, the instrument's physiological sub-scale shows poorer psychometric properties than the fear and avoidance sub-scales and should be used with caution.

Scoring

Part I rates fear in 7 social situations on a 5-point scale ranging from 0 (none) to 4 (extreme – incapacitating and/or very painfully distressing) and avoidance on a 5-point scale ranging from 0 (never – 0%) to 4 (always – 100%). Part II asks the clinician to rate the severity of 4 physiological symptoms on a 5-point scale ranging from 0 (none) through to 4 (extreme, incapacitating and/or very painfully distressing). A total score (range 0–72) is derived by summing all items and the BPRS yields 3 sub-scales

(fear, avoidance and physiological arousal). A total score of >20 indicates phobic symptoms of a severity that warrants treatment.

Versions

A computerized version is available, as is a clinical interactive voice response (IVR) version from Healthcare Technology Systems, Inc.

Additional references

Clark DB, Feske U, Masia CL, Spaulding SA, Brown C, Mammen O, Shear MK. Systematic assessment of social phobia in clinical practice. Depress Anxiety 1997; 6:47–61.

Davidson JR, Miner CM, De Veaugh-Geiss J, Tupler LA, Colket JT, Potts NL. The Brief Social Phobia Scale: a psychometric evaluation. Psychol Med 1997; 27(1):161–6.

Van Ameringen MA, Lane RM, Walker JR, Bowen RC, Chokka PR, Goldner EM, Johnston DG, Lavallee YJ, Nandy S, Pecknold JC, Hadrava V, Swinson RP. Sertraline treatment of generalized social phobia: a 20–week, double-blind, placebo-controlled study. Am J Psychiatry 2001; 158:275–81.

Address for correspondence

Dr. Jonathan R.T. Davidson
Anxiety and Traumatic Stress Program
Department of Psychiatry and Behavioral Sciences
Duke University Medical Center
Trent Drive, Fourth Floor, Yellow 4082B, Box 3812
Durham, NC 27710, USA
Telephone: 1-919-684-2880
Email: jonathan.davidson@duke.edu

Brief Social Phobia Scale (BSPS)

Instructions: The time period will cover the previous week, unless otherwise specified (e.g. at the initial evaluation interview, when it could be the previous month).

Part I. (Fear/Avoidance)

How much do you fear and avoid the following situations? Please give separate ratings for fear and avoidance.

	Fear Rating	Avoidance Rating
	0 = None	0 = Never
	1 = Mild	1 = Rare
	2 = Moderate	2 = Sometimes
	3 = Severe	3 = Frequent
	4 = Extreme	4 = Always
	Fear (F)	Avoidance (A)
1. Speaking in public or in front of others	_____	_____
2. Talking to people in authority	_____	_____
3. Talking to strangers	_____	_____
4. Being embarrassed or humiliated	_____	_____
5. Being criticized	_____	_____
6. Social gathering	_____	_____
7. Doing something while being watched (this does not include speaking)	_____	_____

Part II. Physiologic (P)

When you are in a situation that involves contact with other people, or when you are thinking about such a situation, do you experience the following symptoms?

	0 = None
	1 = Mild
	2 = Moderate
	3 = Severe
	4 = Extreme
8. Blushing	_____
9. Palpitations	_____
10. Trembling	_____
11. Sweating	_____

Total scores: F = _____   A = _____   P = _____   Total = _____

Clinician-Administered PTSD Scale (CAPS)

Reference: **Blake DD, Weathers FW, Nagy LM, Kaloupek DG, Klauminzer G, Charney DS, Keane TM. A clinician rating scale for assessing current and lifetime PTSD: The CAPS-I. Behav Ther 1990; 13:187–8**

Rating Clinician-rated

Administration time 45–60 minutes

Main purpose To diagnose and assess severity of PTSD symptoms

Population Adults and adolescents

Commentary

The CAPS is a comprehensive structured clinical interview designed to assess the 17 symptoms of PTSD (current, lifetime or during the past week) outlined in DSM-III-R (or modified for DSM-IV) along with 5 associated features (guilt, dissociation, derealization, depersonalization, and reduction in awareness of surroundings). The instrument contains a checklist of potentially traumatizing events, of which up to 3 may be selected based on their severity or recency. A description of the events is obtained by the clinician, as well as details of the patient's emotional response to the events in order to establish DSM-IV criterion A for PTSD. Following this, DSM-IV criterion B (e.g. flashbacks, dreams, recurrent and intrusive thoughts), criterion C (e.g. avoidance, restricted affect) and criterion D (symptoms of increased arousal such as sleep problems or poor concentration) are evaluated. Criterion E is assessed via 2 questions concerning onset and duration of symptoms and Criterion F by 3 items addressing distress and impairment in functioning. Although the CAPS was originally developed for use in military personnel, it is appropriate for use in civilian populations. Whilst generally too lengthy to be used as a screening tool, the CAPS is currently the standard criterion measure in the field of traumatic stress and represents a reliable and valid method for diagnosing PTSD, assessing baseline severity of symptoms and response to treatment.

Scoring

Items are rated for frequency on a 5-point scale from 0 (never) through to 4 (daily or almost every day) and intensity, on a scale from 0 (none) through to 4 (extreme). A total score (range 0–136) can be obtained by summing the frequency and intensity scores for each of the 17 items, and the CAPS can provide a dichotomous rating for the presence or absence of PTSD.

Versions

A child and adolescent version of the CAPS is available via the National Centre for PTSD website (http://www.ncptsd.org). The scale has been translated into French, German, Japanese, Russian and Spanish.

Additional references

Blake DD, Weathers FW, Nagy LM, Kaloupek DG, Gusman FD, Charney DS, Keane TM. The development of a Clinician-Administered PTSD Scale. J Trauma Stress 1995; 8(1):75–90

Weathers FW, Keane TM, Davidson JR. Clinician-administered PTSD scale: a review of the first ten years of research. Depress Anxiety 2001; 13(3):132–56.

Address for correspondence

National Center for PTSD (116D)
VA Medical Center & Regional Office Center
215 North Main St.
White River Junction, VT 05009, USA
Telephone: 1-802-296-6300
Email: ncptsd@ncptsd.org

Clinician-Administered PTSD Scale – sample items

Have you ever suddenly acted or felt as if the event was happening again? How often in the past month?

At its worst, how much did it seem that the event was happening again? How long did it last? What did you do while this was happening?

Reproduced from Blake DD, Weathers FW, Nagy LM, et al. Behav Ther 1990; 13:187–8 with permission from the National Center for PTSD, www.ncptsd.org.

Covi Anxiety Scale (COVI)

Reference: **Lipman RS. Differentiating anxiety and depression in anxiety disorders: use of rating scales. Psychopharmacol Bull 1982; 18(4):69–77**

Rating Clinician-rated

Administration time 5–10 minutes

Main purpose To assess severity of symptoms of anxiety

Population Adults

Commentary

The COVI is a simple 3-item clinician-rated scale that assesses severity of anxiety in terms of the patient's verbal report, behaviour and somatic symptoms. Although there is relatively little extant data concerning the scale's psychometric properties, it has been widely used as an inclusion/exclusion criteria and outcome measure in pharmaceutical trials.

Scoring

Items are rated on a 5-point scale ranging from 1 (not at all) through to 5 (very much).

Versions

No other versions available.

Additional references

Lipman RS, Covi L, Downing RW. Pharmacotherapy of anxiety and depression. Psychopharmacol Bull 1981; 17(3):91–103.

Chouinard G, Saxena B, Belanger MC, Ravindran A, Bakish D, Beauclair L, Morris P, Vasavan Nair NP, Manchanda R, Reesal R, Remick R, O'Neill MC. A Canadian multicenter, double-blind study of paroxetine and fluoxetine in major depressive disorder. J Affect Disord 1999; 54(1–2):39–48.

Silverstone PH, Salinas E. Efficacy of venlafaxine extended release in patients with major depressive disorder and comorbid generalized anxiety disorder. J Clin Psychiatry 2001; 62(7):523–9.

Address for correspondence

None available

COVI Anxiety Scale

Rate each of the following according to the degrees of severity below:

1 = not at all; 2 = somewhat; 3 = moderately; 4 = considerably; 5 = very much

I. _____ Verbal report: Feels nervous, shaky, jittery, suddenly fearful or scared for no reason, tense, has to avoid certain situations, places, or things because of getting frightened, difficulty in concentrating

II. _____ Behavior: Looks scared, shaking, apprehensive, restless, jittery

III. _____ Somatic symptoms of anxiety: Trembling, sweating, rapid heartbeat, breathlessness, hot or cold spells, restless sleep, discomfort in stomach, lump in throat, having to go to the bathroom frequently

Reproduced from Lipman RS. Psychopharmacol Bull 1982; 18(4):69–77.

Davidson Trauma Scale (DTS)

Reference: **Davidson JR, Book SW, Colket JT, Tupler LA, Roth S, David D, Hertzberg M, Mellman T, Beckham JC, Smith RD, Davison RM, Katz R, Feldman ME. Assessment of a new self-rating scale for post-traumatic stress disorder. Psychol Med 1997; 27(1):153–60**

Rating Self-report

Administration time 10 minutes

Main purpose To assess symptoms of PTSD

Population Adults

Commentary

A 17-item self-report scale that reflects DSM-IV criteria, the DTS was designed to assess severity of PTSD symptoms from all types of trauma, such as sexual/criminal assault, combat, injury or bereavement. The scale yields 3 sub-scales: intrusion, avoidance/numbing and hyperarousal. Respondents are asked to rate each of the 17 items referring to a particular traumatic event, or series of events, for both frequency and severity over the past week. If the respondent has experienced several traumatic episodes, multiple copies of the DTS may be administered. The DTS is appropriate for both screening for PTSD and monitoring response to treatment. A 4-item scale called the SPAN (Startle, Physiological arousal, Anger and Numbness) has been developed from the DTS, providing an even briefer screening instrument.

Scoring

Items are scored on a 5-point scale for both frequency (from 0, not at all, through to 4, every day) and severity (from 0, not at all distressing, through to 4, extremely distressing). A total score is derived by summing all the items; sub-scale scores can be calculated for frequency, severity and for each of the 3 symptom clusters.

Versions

The DTS has been translated into Chinese, French-Canadian and Spanish. A computer-administered version is available.

Additional references

Meltzer-Brody S, Churchill E, Davidson JR. Derivation of the SPAN, a brief diagnostic screening test for post-traumatic stress disorder. Psychiatry Res 1999; 88(1):63–70.

Davidson JR, Tharwani HM, Connor KM. Davidson Trauma Scale (DTS): normative scores in the general population and effect sizes in placebo-controlled SSRI trials. Depress Anxiety 2002; 15(2):75–8.

Address for correspondence

Multi-Health Systems Inc.
P.O. Box 950
North Tonawanda, NY 14120–0950, USA
Telephone: 1-800-456-3003 in the US or
1-416-492-2627 international
Email: customerservice@mhs.com
Website: www.mhs.com

Depression Anxiety Stress Scales (DASS)

Reference: Lovibond SH, Lovibond, PF. Manual for the Depression Anxiety Stress Scales. 1995. Sydney, NSW, The Psychology Foundation of Australia

Rating Self-report

Administration time 10 minutes

Main purpose To detect core symptoms of depression, anxiety and stress using a dimensional approach

Population Adults and adolescents

Commentary

The DASS is a 42-item self-report scale developed to assess symptoms of depression, anxiety and stress/tension over the previous week. The instrument possesses 3 scales: depression (D), anxiety (A) and stress (S), each of which has 14 items, further divided into subscales of 2–5 items with similar content. The instrument provides a useful method for concomitantly assessing symptoms of depression, anxiety and tension, whilst allowing the clinician to discriminate between these constructs. The scale developers state that the principal clinical value of the DASS is to clarify the locus of emotional disturbance, as part of the broader task of clinical assessment; it has not been used extensively to monitor treatment response. An abbreviated 21-item form with 7 items per scale (DASS21) is also available, and takes approximately 5 minutes to administer.

Scoring

Items are scored on a 0–3 scale, scores for the D, A and S scales are derived by summing the items in each scale (range 0–42). For the D scale, scores of 0–9 are in the normal range; 10–13, mild; 14–20, moderate; 21–27, severe; ≥28, very severe. For the A scale, scores of 0–7 are considered normal; 8–9, mild; 10–14, moderate; 15–19, severe; ≥20, very severe. For the S scale, scores of 0–14 are normal; 15–18, mild; 19–25, moderate; 26–33, severe; ≥34, very severe.

Versions

The DASS has been translated into Arabic, Chinese, Dutch, Hungarian, Japanese, Persian, Spanish and Vietnamese.

Additional references

Lovibond PF, Lovibond SH. The structure of negative emotional states: comparison of the Depression Anxiety Stress Scales (DASS) with the Beck Depression and Anxiety Inventories. Behav Res Ther 1995; 33(3):335–43.

Antony MM, Bieling PJ, Cox BJ, Enns MW, Swinson RP. Psychometric properties of the 42-item and 21-item versions of the Depression Anxiety Stress Scales (DASS) in clinical groups and a community sample. Psychol Assess 1998; 10:176–81.

Nieuwenhuijsen K, de Boer AG, Verbeek JH, Blonk RW, van Dijk FJ. The Depression Anxiety Stress Scales (DASS): detecting anxiety disorder and depression in employees absent from work because of mental health problems. Occup Environ Med 2003; 60 (Suppl 1): 177–82.

Address for correspondence

Professor Peter Lovibond
School of Psychology
University of New South Wales
Sydney, NSW 2052, Australia
Telephone: 61-2-9385 3034
Email: P.Lovibond@unsw.edu.au
Website: http://www.psy.unsw.edu.au/Groups/Dass/

DASS

Please read each statement and circle a number 0, 1, 2 or 3 which indicates how much the statement applied to you *over the past week*. There are no right or wrong answers. Do not spend too much time on any statement.

The rating scale is as follows:

0   Did not apply to me at all
1   Applied to me to some degree, or some of the time
2   Applied to me to a considerable degree, or a good part of the time
3   Applied to me very much, or most of the time

1	I found myself getting upset by quite trivial things	0	1	2	3
2	I was aware of dryness of my mouth	0	1	2	3
3	I couldn't seem to experience any positive feeling at all	0	1	2	3
4	I experienced breathing difficulty (e.g., excessively rapid breathing, breathlessness in the absence of physical exertion)	0	1	2	3
5	I just couldn't seem to get going	0	1	2	3
6	I tended to over-react to situations	0	1	2	3
7	I had a feeling of shakiness (e.g., legs going to give way)	0	1	2	3
8	I found it difficult to relax	0	1	2	3
9	I found myself in situations that made me so anxious I was most relieved when they ended	0	1	2	3
10	I felt that I had nothing to look forward to	0	1	2	3
11	I found myself getting upset rather easily	0	1	2	3
12	I felt that I was using a lot of nervous energy	0	1	2	3
13	I felt sad and depressed	0	1	2	3
14	I found myself getting impatient when I was delayed in any way (e.g., lifts, traffic lights, being kept waiting)	0	1	2	3
15	I had a feeling of faintness	0	1	2	3
16	I felt that I had lost interest in just about everything	0	1	2	3
17	I felt I wasn't worth much as a person	0	1	2	3
18	I felt that I was rather touchy	0	1	2	3
19	I perspired noticeably (e.g., hands sweaty) in the absence of high temperatures or physical exertion	0	1	2	3
20	I felt scared without any good reason	0	1	2	3
21	I felt that life wasn't worthwhile	0	1	2	3
22	I found it hard to wind down	0	1	2	3
23	I had difficulty in swallowing	0	1	2	3
24	I couldn't seem to get any enjoyment out of the things I did	0	1	2	3
25	I was aware of the action of my heart in the absence of physical exertion (e.g., sense of heart rate increase, heart missing a beat)	0	1	2	3
26	I felt down-hearted and blue	0	1	2	3
27	I found that I was very irritable	0	1	2	3
28	I felt I was close to panic	0	1	2	3
29	I found it hard to calm down after something upset me	0	1	2	3
30	I feared that I would be "thrown" by some trivial but unfamiliar task	0	1	2	3
31	I was unable to become enthusiastic about anything	0	1	2	3
32	I found it difficult to tolerate interruptions to what I was doing	0	1	2	3
33	I was in a state of nervous tension	0	1	2	3
34	I felt I was pretty worthless	0	1	2	3
35	I was intolerant of anything that kept me from getting on with what I was doing	0	1	2	3
36	I felt terrified	0	1	2	3
37	I could see nothing in the future to be hopeful about	0	1	2	3
38	I felt that life was meaningless	0	1	2	3
39	I found myself getting agitated	0	1	2	3
40	I was worried about situations in which I might panic and make a fool of myself	0	1	2	3
41	I experienced trembling (e.g., in the hands)	0	1	2	3
42	I found it difficult to work up the initiative to do things	0	1	2	3

DASS can be downloaded without charge as above or as a short (21 item) version from www.psy.unsw.edu.au/dass/.

Fear of Negative Evaluation Scale (FNE) and Social Avoidance and Distress Scale (SADS)

Reference: **Watson D, Friend R. Measurement of social-evaluative anxiety. J Consult Clin Psychol 1969; 33(4):448–57**

Rating Self-report

Administration time 10 minutes each

Main purpose To assess fear of social evaluation and distress and avoidance in social situations

Population Adults

Commentary

The FNE and the SAD were designed as complementary self-report measures of social anxiety to be used together. The FNE is a 30-item instrument developed to assess expectations and distress associated with negative evaluation by others. The SAD is a 28-item scale that measures two aspects of anxiety; an individual's experience of distress in social situations, and avoidance of social situations. Both instruments have shown the ability to differentiate between patients with social phobia and those with simple (specific) phobia. There is some question, however, of whether they can differentiate social phobia from GAD or panic disorder (Oei et al., 1991).

Scoring

Both scales are scored in a true/false format, with higher scores indicating greater social anxiety.

Versions

The SAD has been translated into Chinese, German, Hindi, Japanese and Swedish. The FNE has been translated into Japanese. A brief 12-item version of the FNE has been developed.

Additional references

Turner SM, McCanna M, Beidel DC. Validity of the Social Avoidance and Distress and Fear of Negative Evaluation Scale. Behav Res Ther 1987; 25:113–15.

Heimberg RG, Hope DA, Rapee RM, Bruch MA. The validity of the Social Avoidance and Distress Scale and the Fear of Negative Evaluation Scale with social phobic patients. Behav Res Ther 1988; 26(5):407–13.

Oei TP, Kenna D, Evans L. The reliability, validity, and utility of the SAD and FNE scales for anxiety disorder patients. Pers Individ Dif 1991; 12:111–16.

Address for correspondence

Dr. Ronald Friend
2347 NW Overton St.
Portland, OR 97210, USA
Telephone: 1-503-241-1881
Email: Ronald.Friend@sunysb.edu

Social Avoidance and Distress Scale (SADS)

For the following statements, please answer each in terms of whether it is true or false for you.
Circle T for true or F for false.

T	F	1.	I feel relaxed even in unfamiliar social situations.
T	F	2.	I try to avoid situations which force me to be very sociable.
T	F	3.	It is easy for me to relax when I am with strangers.
T	F	4.	I have no particular desire to avoid people.
T	F	5.	I often find social occasions upsetting.
T	F	6.	I usually feel calm and comfortable at social occasions.
T	F	7.	I am usually at ease when talking to someone of the opposite sex.
T	F	8.	I try to avoid talking to people unless I know them well.
T	F	9.	If the chance comes to meet new people, I often take it.
T	F	10.	I often feel nervous or tense in casual get-togethers in which both sexes are present.
T	F	11.	I am usually nervous with people unless I know them well.
T	F	12.	I usually feel relaxed when I am with a group of people.
T	F	13.	I often want to get away from people.
T	F	14.	I usually feel uncomfortable when I am in a group of people I don't know.
T	F	15.	I usually feel relaxed when I meet someone for the first time.
T	F	16.	Being introduced to people makes me tense and nervous.
T	F	17.	Even though a room is full of strangers, I may enter it anyway.
T	F	18.	I would avoid walking up and joining a large group of people.
T	F	19.	When my superiors want to talk with me, I talk willingly.
T	F	20.	I often feel on edge when I am with a group of people,
T	F	21.	I tend to withdraw from people.
T	F	22.	I don't mind talking to people at parties or social gatherings.
T	F	23.	I am seldom at ease in a large group of people.
T	F	24.	I often think up excuses in order to avoid social engagements.
T	F	25.	I sometimes take the responsibility for introducing people to each other.
T	F	26.	I try to avoid formal social occasions.
T	F	27.	I usually go to whatever social engagement I have.
T	F	28.	I find it easy to relax with other people.

Reprinted from Watson, D and Friend, R. *J Consult Clin Psychol* 1969; 33:448–57. Copyright © 1969 by the American Psychological Association. Reprinted with permission.

Fear of Negative Evaluation Scale (FNE)

For the following statements, please answer each in terms of whether it is true or false for you.
Circle T for true or F for false.

T	F	1.	I rarely worry about seeming foolish to others.
T	F	2.	I worry about what people will think of me even when I know it doesn't make any difference.
T	F	3.	I become tense and jittery if I know someone is sizing me up.
T	F	4.	I am unconcerned even if I know people are forming an unfavorable impression of me.
T	F	5.	I feel very upset when I commit some social error.
T	F	6.	The opinions that important people have of me cause me little concern.
T	F	7.	I am often afraid that I may look ridiculous or make a fool of myself.
T	F	8.	I react very little when other people disapprove of me.
T	F	9.	I am frequently afraid of other people noticing my shortcomings.
T	F	10.	The disapproval of others would have little effect on me.
T	F	11.	If someone is evaluating me I tend to expect the worst.
T	F	12.	I rarely worry about what kind of impression I am making on someone.
T	F	13.	I am afraid that others will not approve of me.
T	F	14.	I am afraid that people will find fault with me.
T	F	15.	Other people's opinions of me do not bother me.
T	F	16.	I am not necessarily upset if I do not please someone.
T	F	17.	When I am talking to someone, I worry about what they may be thinking about me.
T	F	18.	I feel that you can't help making social errors sometimes, so why worry about it.
T	F	19.	I am usually worried about what kind of impression I make.
T	F	20.	I worry a lot about what my superiors think of me.
T	F	21.	If I know someone is judging me, it has little effect on me.
T	F	22.	I worry that others will think I am not worthwhile.
T	F	23.	I worry very little about what others may think of me.
T	F	24.	Sometimes I think I am too concerned with what other people think of me.
T	F	25.	I often worry that I will say or do the wrong things.
T	F	26.	I am often indifferent to the opinions others have of me.
T	F	27.	I am usually confident that others will have a favorable impression of me.
T	F	28.	I often worry that people who are important to me won't think very much of me.
T	F	29.	I brood about the opinions my friends have about me.
T	F	30.	I become tense and jittery if I know I am being judged by my superiors.

Reprinted from Watson, D and Friend, R. *J Consult Clin Psychol* 1969; 33:448–57. Copyright © 1969 by the American Psychological Association.
Reprinted with permission.

Fear Questionnaire (FQ)

Reference: **Marks IM, Mathews AM. Brief standard self-rating for phobic patients. Behav Res Ther 1979; 17(3):263–7**

Rating Self-report

Administration time 10 minutes

Main purpose To measure severity of, and change in, common phobias and related anxiety and depression

Population Adults

Commentary

The FQ is a frequently used 24-item self-report measure designed to assess severity of common phobias, change in phobic symptoms and associated depression and anxiety. The instrument's Total Phobia scale (the most frequently cited score) contains 15 items and yields 3 sub-scales (agoraphobia, blood-injury phobia and social phobia). The scale also provides a 1-item Global Phobic Distress index and a 5-item Anxiety/Depression sub-scale. The agoraphobia and social phobia sub-scales of the FQ are most commonly utilized, and are able to discriminate between patients with panic disorder with agoraphobia and those with social phobia (Cox et al., 1991). The FQ anxiety/depression sub-scale may provide some useful additional data, but is likely to tap general distress rather than serving as a sensitive measure of either disorder. The instrument has been shown to be sensitive to response to treatment in a variety of clinical settings, and was the initial gold standard in the assessment of social phobia.

Scoring

Items are scored on a 9-point scale ranging from 0 (would not avoid it) through to 8 (always avoid it). The total phobia score (FQ-TOT, range 0–120) is obtained by summing responses to items 2 through 16. Sub-scale scores (range 0–40) are derived by simply summing the appropriate items.

Versions

The FQ has been translated into Catalan, Chinese, Dutch, French, German, Italian and Spanish.

Additional references

Cox BJ, Swinson RP, Shaw BF. Value of the Fear Questionnaire in differentiating agoraphobia and social phobia. Br J Psychiatry 1991; 159:842–5.

Oei TPS, Moylan A, Evans L. Validity and clinical utility of the Fear Questionnaire for anxiety-disorder patients. Psychol Assess 1991; 3:391–7.

Cox BJ, Parker JD, Swinson RP. Confirmatory factor analysis of the Fear Questionnaire with social phobia patients. Br J Psychiatry 1996; 168(4):497–9.

Address for correspondence

Dr. Isaac Marks
Department of Psychiatry
Charing Cross Campus
Imperial College London University
303 North End Rd, London W14 9NS, UK
Telephone: +44 (0)20 7610 2594
Email: i.marks@imperial.ac.uk

Fear Questionnaire

Name _____ Age _____ Sex _____ Date _____

Choose a number from the scale below to show how much you would avoid each of the situations listed below because of fear or other unpleasant feelings. Then write the number you chose in the box opposite each situation.

0	1	2	3	4	5	6	7	8
Would not avoid it		Slightly avoid it		Definitely avoid it		Markedly avoid it		Always avoid it

1. Main phobia you want treated (describe in your own words) ☐
2. Injections or minor surgery ☐
3. Eating or drinking with other people ☐
4. Hospitals ☐
5. Travelling alone by bus or coach ☐
6. Walking alone in busy streets ☐
7. Being watched or stared at ☐
8. Going into crowded shops ☐
9. Talking to people in authority ☐
10. Sight of blood ☐
11. Being criticized ☐
12. Going alone far from home ☐
13. Thought of injury or illness ☐
14. Speaking or acting to an audience ☐
15. Large open spaces ☐
16. Going to the dentist ☐
17. Other situations (describe) ☐

Leave blank – ☐☐☐   ☐
Ag + Bl + Soc = Total
2–16

Now choose a number from the scale below to show how much you are troubled by each problem listed, and write the number in the box opposite

0	1	2	3	4	5	6	7	8
Hardly at all		Slightly troublesome		Definitely troublesome		Markedly troublesome		Very severely troublesome

18. Feeling miserable or depressed ☐
19. Feeling irritable or angry ☐
20. Feeling tense or panicky ☐
21. Upsetting thoughts coming into your mind ☐
22. Feeling you or your surroundings are strange or unreal ☐
23. Other feelings (describe) ☐

☐ Total

How would you rate the present state of your phobic symptoms on the scale below?

0	1	2	3	4	5	6	7	8
No phobias present		Slightly disturbing/ not really disabling		Definitely disturbing/ disabling		Markedly disturbing/ disabling		Very severely disturbing/ disabling

Please circle one number between 0 and 8

Reproduced from Marks IM, Mathews AM. Behav Res Ther 1979; 17(3):263–7 with permission from Dr. Isaac Marks. © 1979 Isaac Marks.

Hospital Anxiety and Depression Scale (HADS)

Reference: **Zigmond AS, Snaith RP. The Hospital Anxiety and Depression Scale. Acta Psychiatr Scand 1983; 67(6):361–70**

Rating Self-report

Administration time <5 minutes

Main purpose To screen for depression and anxiety in medical patients

Population Adults, adolescents aged over 16 and older adults

Commentary

The HADS is a 14-item self-report instrument designed to screen for presence and severity of symptoms of depression and anxiety over the past week in medical patients. The instrument possesses a 7-item depression sub-scale (HADS-D) and a 7-item anxiety sub-scale (HADS-A), both of which omit somatic symptoms in an attempt to reduce the likelihood of false-positive diagnoses. The HADS-D concentrates on assessing loss of hedonic tone, which the scale developers' state is a type of depression that is often biological in origin and therefore likely to respond to antidepressant medication. The HADS represents a brief and useful screening tool for symptoms of depression and anxiety in patients with physical illness. Two review articles have further indicated that it is sensitive to change, and that it is appropriate for use in primary care and general population samples.

Scoring

Items are scored on a 0–3 scale: HADS-D and HADS-A sub-scale scores (range 0–21) are derived by summing the 7 items on each scale (the scale developers warn against deriving a total score for the HADS). For both sub-scales, scores in the range of 0–7 are considered normal; 8–10, mild, 11–14, moderate; 15–21, severe.

Versions

The HADS has been translated into: Arabic, Cantonese, Danish, Dutch, French, German, Hebrew, Italian, Japanese, Norwegian, Spanish and Swedish, amongst other languages – contact nferNelson for further details.

Additional references

Herrmann C. International experience with the Hospital Anxiety and Depression Scale. A review of validation data and clinical results. J Psychosom Res 1997; 42:17–41.

Crawford JR, Henry JD, Crombie C, Taylor EP. Normative data for the HADS from a large non-clinical sample. Br J Clin Psychol 2001; 40(Pt 4):429–34.

Bjelland I, Dahl AA, Haug TT, Neckelmann D. The validity of the Hospital Anxiety and Depression Scale; an updated review. J Psychiat Res 2002; 52:69–77.

Address for correspondence

nferNelson
The Chiswick Centre
414 Chiswick High Road
London W4 5TF, UK
Telephone: +44 (0) 20 8996 8444
Email: information@nfer-nelson.co.uk
Website: http://www.nfer-nelson.co.uk

Impact of Event Scale–Revised (IES-R)

Reference: Weiss DS, Marmar CR. The Impact of Event Scale – Revised. In J Wilson, TM Keane (Eds.) Assessing Psychological Trauma and PTSD (pp. 399–411). 1996. New York: Guilford

Rating Self-report

Administration time 5–10 minutes

Main purpose To assess distress (intrusion, avoidance and hyperarousal) associated with stressful life events

Population Adults and adolescents

Commentary

The IES-R is a 22-item self-report measure designed to assess current subjective distress for any specific life event. It replaces the original 15-item Impact of Event Scale (Horowitz et al., 1979) in that it is constructed to parallel DSM-IV criteria for PTSD. The patient is asked to think of a specific stressful event and rate any difficulties the event has caused over the past week. Because the wording of the scale is not event-specific, it can be used to assess a variety of stressful or traumatic events, and is not restricted to use in PTSD populations. Although the instrument yields 3 sub-scales (intrusion, avoidance and hyperarousal), a recent publication reporting a factor analysis of the IES-R provides evidence for a single, or a two-factor solution (intrusion/hyperarousal and avoidance).

Scoring

Items are scored on a 0 (not at all) to 4 (extremely) scale, yielding a total score with a range of 0–88. Sub-scale scores are derived by calculating the mean of the appropriate items.

Versions

The IES-R has been translated into Chinese, French and Japanese.

Additional references

Horowitz M, Wilner N, Alvarez W. Impact of Event Scale: a measure of subjective stress. Psychosom Med 1979; 41(3):209–218.

Creamer M, Bell R, Failla S. Psychometric properties of the Impact of Event Scale – Revised. Behav Res Ther 2003; 41(12):1489–96.

Address for correspondence

Dr. Daniel Weiss
Department of Psychiatry
University of California – San Francisco
Box F-0984
San Francisco, CA 94143-0984, USA
Telephone: 1-415-476-7557
Email: dweiss@itsa.ucsf.edu

Impact of Event Scale–Revised (IES-R)

INSTRUCTIONS: Below is a list of difficulties people sometimes have after stressful life events. Please read each item, and then indicate how distressing each difficulty has been for you **DURING THE PAST SEVEN DAYS** with respect to _____. How much were you distressed or bothered by these difficulties?

Item Response Anchors are 0 = Not at all; 1 = A little bit; 2 = Moderately; 3 = Quite a bit; 4 = Extremely.

The intrusion subscale is the **MEAN** item response of items 1, 2, 3, 6, 9, 14, 16, 20. Thus, scores can range from 0 through 4.

The Avoidance subscale is the **MEAN** item response of items 5, 7, 8, 11, 12, 13, 17, 22. Thus, scores can range from 0 through 4.

The Hyperarousal subscale is the **MEAN** item response of items 4, 10, 15, 18, 19, 21, Thus, scores can range from 0 through 4.

1. Any reminder brought back feelings about it.
2. I had trouble staying asleep.
3. Other things kept making me think about it.
4. I felt irritable and angry.
5. I avoided letting myself get upset when I thought about it or was reminded of it.
6. I thought about it when I didn't mean to.
7. I felt as if it hadn't happened or wasn't real.
8. I stayed away from reminders of it.
9. Pictures about it popped into my mind.
10. I was jumpy and easily startled.
11. I tried not to think about it.
12. I was aware that I still had a lot of feelings about it, but I didn't deal with them.
13. My feelings about it were kind of numb.
14. I found myself acting or feeling like I was back at that time.
15. I had trouble falling asleep.
16. I had waves of strong feelings about it.
17. I tried to remove it from my memory.
18. I had trouble concentrating.
19. Reminders of it caused me to have physical reactions, such as sweating, trouble breathing, nausea, or a pounding heart.
20. I had dreams about it.
21. I felt watchful and on guard.
22. I tried not to talk about it.

Reproduced from Weiss DS, Marmar CR. The Impact of Event Scale – Revised. In J Wilson, TM Keane (Eds.) Assessing Psychological Trauma and PTSD (pp. 399–411). 1996. New York: Guilford with permission from Dr. Daniel Weiss.

Liebowitz Social Anxiety Scale (LSAS)

Reference: **Liebowitz MR. Social phobia. Mod Probl Pharmacopsychiatry 1987; 22:141–73**

Rating Clinician-administered (LSAS) and self-report (LSAS-SR)

Administration time 20–30 minutes

Main purpose To measure fear and avoidance in patients with social phobia

Population Adults

Commentary

The LSAS (sometimes referred to as the Liebowitz Social Phobia Scale or LSPS) is a popular 24-item clinician or self-administered scale designed to measure fear and avoidance in patients with social phobia. The instrument contains 2 sub-scales: social interaction (11 items) and performance (13 items). The LSAS is one of two clinician-administered instruments for assessing social phobia (the other being the more concise Brief Social Phobia Scale or BSPS, see page 69). The LSAS appears to be a relatively reliable, valid and treatment sensitive measure of social phobia (Heimberg et al., 1999), although some studies have found the fear and avoidance ratings for the scale to be highly intercorrelated. The scale has been used extensively in pharmacotherapy research for social phobia. Although the LSAS does not assess cognitive and physiological symptoms and the BSPS does not assess physiological symptoms in depth, either scale can be used clinically to assess severity and change during treatment.

Scoring

Fear items are rated on a 4-point scale ranging from 0 (none) to 3 (severe); avoidance items are rated on a 4-point scale ranging from 0 (never) to 3 (usually). The LSAS provides an overall social anxiety severity rating, and the social interaction and performance sub-scales can be further divided into 4 sub-scales: performance fear, performance avoidance, social fear, and social avoidance. A cut-off score of 30 on the scale's total score has been suggested when using the instrument to screen for social anxiety disorder.

Versions

A child and adolescent version of the scale has been developed (the LSAS-CA), and the scale has been translated into French, Hebrew and Spanish. A clinical interactive voice response (IVR) version is available from Healthcare Technology Systems, Inc.

Additional references

Heimberg RG, Horner KJ, Juster HR, Safren SA, Brown EJ, Schneier FR, Liebowitz MR. Psychometric properties of the Liebowitz Social Anxiety Scale. Psychol Med 1999; 29(1):199–212.

Fresco DM, Coles ME, Heimberg RG, Liebowitz MR, Hami S, Stein MB, Goetz D. The Liebowitz Social Anxiety Scale: a comparison of the psychometric properties of self-report and clinician-administered formats. Psychol Med 2001; 31(6):1025–35

Mennin DS, Fresco DM, Heimberg RG, Schneier FR, Davies SO, Liebowitz MR. Screening for social anxiety disorder in the clinical setting: using the Liebowitz Social Anxiety Scale. J Anxiety Disord 2002; 16(6):661–73.

Address for correspondence

Dr. Michael Liebowitz
New York State Psychiatric Institute
Columbia University
722 West 168th Street
New York, NY 10032, USA
Telephone: 1-212-543-5370
Email: Mrl1945@aol.com

Liebowitz Social Anxiety Scale – sample items

Fear or Anxiety:
0 = None
1 = Mild
2 = Moderate
3 = Severe

Avoidance:
0 = Never (0%)
1 = Occasionally (1–33%)
2 = Often (33–67%)
3 = Usually (67–100%)

	Fear or Anxiety	Avoidance
• Talking to people in authority. (S)		
• Working while being observed. (P)		
• Speaking up at a meeting. (P)		

Maudsley Obsessional Compulsive Inventory (MOCI)

Reference: **Hodgson RS, Rachman S. Obsessional compulsive complaints. Behav Res Ther 1977; 15(5):389–95**

Rating Self-report

Administration time 5 minutes

Main purpose To assess obsessive-compulsive symptoms

Population Adults and adolescents

Commentary

The MOC or MOCI is a 30-item self-report inventory of obsessive-compulsive behaviours and rituals. The MOC's total score shows good psychometric properties, although there have been mixed results in terms of the reliability of the instrument's sub-scales. The instrument was found to reliably discriminate between obsessional patients and normal controls, and between patients with anorexia nervosa versus those with anxiety disorders. It does not, however, appear to discriminate well between patients with OCD and depression (Emmelkamp et al., 1999). The instrument represents a brief, easy-to-administer assessment method for obsessional or compulsive symptoms. A revised version, the Vancouver Obsessional Compulsive Inventory (VOCI) has recently been developed. The VOCI assesses a range of obsessions, compulsions, avoidance behaviours and relevant personality characteristics, and shows promising psychometric properties (Thodarson et al., 2004).

Scoring

Items are scored in true–false manner (0=false, 1=true) with reverse scoring for some items. The scale provides a total score (range 0–30) and 4 sub-scales (checking, cleaning, slowness and doubting).

Versions

The MOC has been translated into Japanese.

Additional references

Sanavio E, Vidotto G. The components of the Maudsley Obsessional-Compulsive Questionnaire. Behav Res Ther 1985; 23(6):659–62.

Emmelkamp PM, Kraaijkamp HJ, van den Hout MA. Assessment of obsessive-compulsive disorder. Behav Modif 1999; 23(2):269–79.

Thordarson DS, Radomsky AS, Rachman S, Shafran R, Sawchuk CN, Hakstian AR. The Vancouver Obsessional Compulsive Inventory (VOCI). Behav Res Ther 2004; 42:1289–314.

Address for correspondence

Dr. Jack Rachman
Department of Psychology
University of British Columbia
1605 – 2136 West Mall
Vancouver, B.C. V6T 1Z4, Canada
Telephone: 1-604-822-5861
Email: rachman@interchange.ubc.ca

Maudsley Obsessional Compulsive Inventory (MOCI)

Please answer each question by putting a circle around the 'T' for True and 'F' for False. There are no right or wrong answers. Work quickly, and do not think too long about the exact meaning of the question.

T   F   1.   I avoid using public telephones because of possible contamination.

T   F   2.   I frequently get nasty thoughts and have difficulty in getting rid of them.

T   F   3.   I am more concerned than most people about honesty.

T   F   4.   I am often late because I can't seem to get through everything on time.

T   F   5.   I don't worry unduly about contamination if I touch an animal.

T   F   6.   I frequently have to check things (e.g., gas or water taps, doors, etc.) several times.

T   F   7.   I have a very strict conscience.

T   F   8.   I find that almost every day I am upset by unpleasant thoughts that come into my mind against my will.

T   F   9.   I do not worry unduly if I accidentally bump into someone.

T   F   10.   I usually have serious doubts about the simple everyday things I do.

T   F   11.   Neither of my parents was very strict during my childhood.

T   F   12.   I tend to get behind in my work because I repeat things over and over again.

T   F   13.   I use only an average amount of soap.

T   F   14.   Some numbers are extremely unlucky.

T   F   15.   I do not check letters over and over again before mailing them.

T   F   16.   I do not take a long time to dress in the morning.

T   F   17.   I am not excessively concerned about cleanliness.

T   F   18.   One of my major problems is that I pay too much attention to detail.

T   F   19.   I can use well-kept toilets without any hesitation.

T   F   20.   My major problem is repeated checking.

T   F   21.   I am not unduly concerned about germs and diseases.

T   F   22.   I do not tend to check things more than once.

T   F   23.   I do not stick to a very strict routine when doing ordinary things.

T   F   24.   My hands do not feel dirty after touching money.

T   F   25.   I do not usually count when doing a routine task.

T   F   26.   I take rather a long time to complete my washing in the morning.

T   F   27.   I do not use a great deal of antiseptics.

T   F   28.   I spend a lot of time every day checking things over and over again.

T   F   29.   Hanging and folding my clothes at night does not take up a lot of time.

T   F   30.   Even when I do something very carefully I often feel that it is not quite right.

Reproduced from Hodgson RS, Rachman S. Behav Res Ther 1977; 15(5):389–95 with permission from Elsevier.

Mobility Inventory for Agoraphobia (MI)

Reference: **Chambless DL, Caputo GC, Jasin SE, Gracely EJ, Williams C. The Mobility Inventory for Agoraphobia. Behav Res Ther 1985; 23(1):35–44**

Rating Self-report

Administration time 10–20 minutes

Main purpose To assess severity of agoraphobic avoidance and frequency of panic attacks

Population Adults

Commentary

The MI is a self-report measure of frequency of panic attacks and agoraphobic avoidance in situations when the patient is either accompanied by another person, or is alone. The scale consists of 4 sections. In the first section, the patient is asked to rate the frequency with which they avoid 26 different situations when alone, and then their level of avoidance when they are accompanied by a trusted companion. The second section of the scale requires that the patient select 5 situations that caused the highest degree of concern or impairment. The third part of the questionnaire evaluates (i) panic frequency over the past week, (ii) panic frequency over the past 3 weeks, and (iii) severity of panic attacks during the past week. The fourth section of the MI assesses the patient's safety zone. Swinson and colleagues (1992) have produced a revised version of the instrument that contains a further sub-scale to rate avoidance 'without medication' to assess possible reliance on medication for coping with phobic situations. In clinical practice, the first section of the MI is often used in isolation. Although the length of the MI may limit its use in some clinical settings, it is probably the best extant assessment tool for agoraphobic avoidance.

Scoring

Items are scored on a 1 (never avoid) to 5 (always avoid) scale. The MI provides 2 sub-scales: avoidance-accompanied (MI-ACC) and avoidance-alone (MI-AAL), obtained by calculating the means for items 1–26 separately for avoidance-alone and items 1–25 for avoidance accompanied (range 1–5). Panic attack frequency is scored as a simple frequency count, and Panic Intensity is scored on a 1–5 Likert-type scale. Other sections (e.g., size of the safety zone) are included solely for treatment planning purposes and are not formally scored.

Versions

The scale has been translated into Dutch, French, German, Greek, Portuguese, Spanish and Swedish.

Additional references

Swinson RP, Cox BJ, Shulman ID, Kuch K, Woszczyna CB. Medication use and the assessment of agoraphobic avoidance. Behav Res Ther 1992; 30(6):563–8.

Cox BJ, Swinson RP, Kuch K, Reichman JT. Dimensions of agoraphobia assessed by the Mobility Inventory. Behav Res Ther 1993; 31(4):427–31.

de Beurs E, Chambless DL, Goldstein AJ. Measurement of panic disorder by a modified panic diary. Depress Anxiety 1997; 6(4):133–9.

Address for correspondence

Dr. Dianne L. Chambless
Department of Psychology
University of Pennsylvania
3720 Walnut Street
Philadelphia, PA 19104-6241, USA
Telephone: 1-215-898-5030
Email: chambless@psych.upenn.edu

Mobility Inventory for Agoraphobia

Client ID _____   Date _____

1. Please indicate the degree to which you avoid the following places or situations because of discomfort or anxiety. Rate your amount of avoidance when you are with a companion and when you are alone. Do this by using the following scale:

1	2	3	4	5
never avoid	rarely avoid	avoid about half of the time	avoid most of the time	always avoid

Circle the number for each situation or place under both conditions: when accompanied and when alone. Leave blank situations that do not apply to you.

Places	When accompanied					When alone				
Theaters	1	2	3	4	5	1	2	3	4	5
Supermarkets	1	2	3	4	5	1	2	3	4	5
Shopping malls	1	2	3	4	5	1	2	3	4	5
Classrooms	1	2	3	4	5	1	2	3	4	5
Department stores	1	2	3	4	5	1	2	3	4	5
Restaurants	1	2	3	4	5	1	2	3	4	5
Museums	1	2	3	4	5	1	2	3	4	5
Elavators	1	2	3	4	5	1	2	3	4	5
Auditoriums or stadiums	1	2	3	4	5	1	2	3	4	5
Garages	1	2	3	4	5	1	2	3	4	5
High places Please tell how high	1	2	3	4	5	1	2	3	4	5
Enclosed places	1	2	3	4	5	1	2	3	4	5

Open spaces	When accompanied					When alone				
Outside (for example: fields, wide streets, courtyards)	1	2	3	4	5	1	2	3	4	5
Inside (for example: large rooms, lobbies)	1	2	3	4	5	1	2	3	4	5

Riding in	When accompanied					When alone				
Buses	1	2	3	4	5	1	2	3	4	5
Trains	1	2	3	4	5	1	2	3	4	5
Subways	1	2	3	4	5	1	2	3	4	5
Airplanes	1	2	3	4	5	1	2	3	4	5
Boats	1	2	3	4	5	1	2	3	4	5

Driving or riding in car	When accompanied					When alone				
A. at anytime	1	2	3	4	5	1	2	3	4	5
B. on expressways	1	2	3	4	5	1	2	3	4	5

Situations	When accompanied					When alone				
Standing in lines	1	2	3	4	5	1	2	3	4	5
Crossing bridges	1	2	3	4	5	1	2	3	4	5
Parties or social gatherings	1	2	3	4	5	1	2	3	4	5
Walking on the street	1	2	3	4	5	1	2	3	4	5
Staying at home alone						1	2	3	4	5
Being far away from home	1	2	3	4	5	1	2	3	4	5
Other (specify):	1	2	3	4	5	1	2	3	4	5

2. After completing the first step, circle the five items with which you are most concerned. Of the items listed, these are the five situations or places where avoidance/anxiety most affects your life in a negative way.

Panic attacks

3. We define a panic attack as:
   1. A high level of anxiety accompanied by ...
   2. strong body reactions (heart palpitations, sweating, muscle tremors, dizziness, nausea) with ...
   3. the temporary loss of the ability to plan, think, or reason and ...
   4. the intense desire to escape or flee the situation. (Note: This is different from high anxiety or fear alone.)
   Please indicate the total number of panic attacks you have had in the last 7 days:
   In the last 3 weeks:
   How severe or intense have the panic attacks been? (Place an X on the line below):

very mild	mild	moderately severe	very severe	extremely severe
1	2	3	4	5

Safety zone

4. Many people are able to travel alone freely in an area (usually around their home) or in their safety zone. Do you have such a zone? If yes, please describe:
   a. its location
   b. its size (e.g. radius from home)

Obsessive Compulsive Inventory (OCI)

Reference: **Foa EB, Kozak MJ, Salkovskis PM, Coles ME, Amir N. The validation of a new obsessive-compulsive disorder scale: The obsessive-compulsive inventory. Psychol Assess 1998; 10(3):206–14**

Rating Self-report

Administration time 15 minutes

Main purpose To assess severity of obsessive-compulsive symptoms

Population Adults

Commentary

The OCI is a relatively new 42-item self-report inventory for determining the diagnosis and severity of obsessive-compulsive disorder. The scale requires that the patient rate both the frequency with which particular obsessions and compulsions occur, and the distress caused by the symptoms. The instrument contains 7 sub-scales: washing, checking, doubting, ordering, obsessing, hoarding and mental neutralizing. A revised brief version of the scale (the OCI-R, reproduced here) that has 18 items and 6 sub-scales has also been developed.

Scoring

For the OCI-R, distress is scored on a 5-point scale ranging from 0 (not at all) to 4 (extremely), yielding a total possible score range of 0–72. Sub-scale scores are derived by calculating the mean of the appropriate items.

Versions

A child version (OCI-CV) of the obsessive-compulsive inventory is also available.

Additional reference

Foa EB, Huppert JD, Leiberg S, Langner R, Kichic R, Hajcak G, Salkovskis PM. The Obsessive-Compulsive Inventory: development and validation of a short version. Psychol Assess 2002; 14(4):485–96.

Address for correspondence

Dr. Edna B. Foa
Center for the Treatment and Study of Anxiety
Department of Psychiatry
University of Pennsylvania School of Medicine
3535 Market Street, 6th Floor
Philadelphia, PA 19104, USA
Telephone: 1-215-746-3327
E-mail: foa@mail.med.upenn.edu

OCI-R

The following statements refer to experiences that many people have in their everyday lives. Circle the number that best describes **HOW MUCH** that experience has **DISTRESSED or BOTHERED you during the PAST MONTH**. The numbers refer to the following verbal labels:

0 = Not at all   3 = A lot
1 = A little   4 = Extremely
2 = Moderately

1.	I have saved up so many things that they get in the way.	0	1	2	3	4
2.	I check things more often than necessary.	0	1	2	3	4
3.	I get upset if objects are not arranged properly.	0	1	2	3	4
4.	I feel compelled to count while I am doing things.	0	1	2	3	4
5.	I find it difficult to touch an object when I know it has been touched by strangers or certain people.	0	1	2	3	4
6.	I find it difficult to control my own thoughts.	0	1	2	3	4
7.	I collect things I don't need.	0	1	2	3	4
8.	I repeatedly check doors, windows, drawers, etc.	0	1	2	3	4
9.	I get upset if others change the way I have arranged things.	0	1	2	3	4
10.	I feel I have to repeat certain numbers.	0	1	2	3	4
11.	I sometimes have to wash or clean myself simply because I feel contaminated.	0	1	2	3	4
12.	I am upset by unpleasant thoughts that come into my mind against my will.	0	1	2	3	4
13.	I avoid throwing things away because I am afraid I might need them later.	0	1	2	3	4
14.	I repeatedly check gas and water taps and light switches after turning them off.	0	1	2	3	4
15.	I need things to be arranged in a particular order.	0	1	2	3	4
16.	I feel that there are good and bad numbers.	0	1	2	3	4
17.	I wash my hands more often and longer than necessary.	0	1	2	3	4
18.	I frequently get nasty thoughts and have difficulty in getting rid of them.	0	1	2	3	4

The total and sub-scale scores are obtained by adding the scores of the respective items.

Reproduced from Foa EB, Huppert JD, Leiberg S, et al. Psychol Assess 2002; 14(4):485–96. © 2002 Edna B Foa.

Padua Inventory–Washington State University Revision (PI-WSUR)

Reference: **Burns GL, Keortge SG, Formea GM, Sternberger LG. Revision of the Padua Inventory of obsessive compulsive disorder symptoms: distinctions between worry, obsessions, and compulsions. Behav Res Ther 1996; 34(2):163–73**

Rating Self-report

Administration time 10 minutes

Main purpose To assess severity of obsessions and compulsions

Population Adults and older adolescents

Commentary

Three versions of the Padua Inventory (PI) have been developed: the original 60-item scale (Sanavio, 1988), the 41-item PI-R (van Oppen et al., 1995) and the version described here, the 39-item PI-WSUR (Burns et al., 1996). The PI-WSUR differs from some other assessment scales for obsessive–compulsive disorder in that it measures both obsessions and compulsions (scales such as the MOCI, see page 86, concentrate on measuring compulsions). The instrument provides 5 sub-scales: contamination obsessions and washing compulsions (COWC), dressing/grooming compulsions (DRGRC), checking compulsions (CHCK), obsessional thoughts of harm to self/others (OTAHSO) and obsessional impulses to harm self/others (OITHSO). Unlike the PI and PI-R, the PI-WSUR shows reasonable ability to discriminate between symptoms of OCD and worry, as measured by the Penn State Worry Questionnaire (see page 102) (Burns et al., 1996). The PI-WSUR currently represents the best available self-report measure for assessing severity of obsessive–compulsive symptoms and monitoring response to treatment.

Scoring

All items are scored on a 0 (not at all) to 4 (very much) scale with a total score range (calculated by summing all items) of 0–156. Scores for the 5 sub-scales are calculated by summing the appropriate items (number of items varies by sub-scale).

Versions

The PI-WSUR has been translated into German, Spanish and Turkish; the original PI is available in a wide range of languages.

Additional references

Sanavio E. Obsessions and compulsions: the Padua Inventory. Behav Res Ther 1988; 26(2):169–77.

Van Oppen P, Hoekstra RJ, Emmelkamp PM. The structure of obsessive-compulsive symptoms. Behav Res Ther 1995; 33(1):15–23.

Address for correspondence

Dr. G. Leonard Burns
Department of Psychology
Washington State University
Pullman, WA 99164-4820, USA
Telephone: 1-509-335-8229
E-mail: glburns@mail.wsu.edu

Padua Inventory–Washington State University Revision

Reference for the revision:
Burns, G.L. (1995). Padua Inventory–Washington State University Revision. Pullman, WA: Author. (Available from G. Leonard Burns, Department of Psychology, Washington State University, Pullman, WA 99164-4820, USA)

Sub-scales:

1. Contamination obsessions and washing compulsions sub-scale:
   Items: 1, 2, 3, 4, 5, 6, 7, 8, 9, 10
2. Dressing/grooming compulsions sub-scale:
   Items: 11, 12, 13.
3. Checking compulsions sub-scale:
   Items: 14, 15, 16, 17, 18, 19, 20, 21, 22, 23
4. Obsessional thoughts of harm to self/others sub-scale:
   Items: 24, 25, 26, 27, 28, 29, 30
5. Obsessional impulses to harm self/others sub-scale:
   Items: 31, 32, 33, 34, 35, 36, 37, 38, 39

Reference for the psychometric properties of the revision:
Burns, G.L., Keortge, S., Formea, G., Stemberger, L.G. (1996). Revision of the Padua Inventory of obsessive compulsive disorder symptoms: Distinctions between worry, obsessions, and compulsions. Behavior Research and Therapy, 34, 163–73.

The following statements refer to thoughts and behaviors which may occur to everyone in everyday life. For each statement, choose the reply which best seems to fit you and the degree of disturbance which such thoughts or behaviors may create.

1	I feel my hands are dirty when I touch money.	Not at All	A little	Quite A Lot	A Lot	Very Much
2	I think even slight contact with bodily secretions (perspiration, saliva, urine, etc.) may contaminate my clothes or somehow harm me.	Not at All	A little	Quite A Lot	A Lot	Very Much
3	I find it difficult to touch an object when I know it has been touched by strangers or by certain people.	Not at All	A little	Quite a Lot	A Lot	Very Much
4	I find it difficult to touch garbage or dirty things.	Not at All	A little	Quite a Lot	A Lot	Very Much
5	I avoid using public toilets because I am afraid of disease and contamination.	Not at All	A little	Quite a Lot	A Lot	Very Much
6	I avoid using public telephones because I am afraid of contagion and disease.	Not at All	A little	Quite a Lot	A Lot	Very Much
7	I wash my hands more often and longer than necessary.	Not at All	A little	Quite a Lot	A Lot	Very Much
8	I sometimes have to wash or clean myself simply because I think I may be dirty or 'contaminated'.	Not at All	A little	Quite a Lot	A Lot	Very Much
9	If I touch something I think is 'contaminated', I immediately have to wash or . clean myself	Not at All	A little	Quite a Lot	A Lot	Very Much
10	If an animal touches me, I feel dirty and immediately have to wash myself or change my clothing.	Not at All	A little	Quite a Lot	A Lot	Very Much
11	I feel obliged to follow a particular order in dressing, undressing, and washing myself.	Not at All	A little	Quite a Lot	A Lot	Very Much
12	Before going to sleep, I have to do certain things in a certain order.	Not at All	A little	Quite a Lot	A Lot	Very Much
13	Before going to bed, I have to hang up or fold my clothes in a special way.	Not at All	A little	Quite a Lot	A Lot	Very Much
14	I have to do things several times before I think they are properly done.	Not at All	A little	Quite a Lot	A Lot	Very Much
15	I tend to keep on checking things more often than necessary.	Not at All	A little	Quite a Lot	A Lot	Very Much
16	I check and recheck gas and water taps and light switches after turning them off.	Not at All	A little	Quite a Lot	A Lot	Very Much
17	I return home to check doors, windows, drawers, etc., to make sure they are properly shut.	Not at All	A little	Quite a Lot	A Lot	Very Much
18	I keep on checking forms, documents, checks, etc., in detail to make sure I have filled them in correctly.	Not at All	A little	Quite a Lot	A Lot	Very Much
19	I keep on going back to see that matches, cigarettes, etc, are properly extinguished.	Not at All	A little	Quite a Lot	A Lot	Very Much
20	When I handle money, I count and recount it several times.	Not at All	A little	Quite a Lot	A Lot	Very Much
21	I check letters carefully many times before posting them.	Not at All	A little	Quite a Lot	A Lot	Very Much
22	Sometimes I am not sure I have done things which in fact I knew I have done.	Not at All	A little	Quite a Lot	A Lot	Very Much
23	When I read, I have the impression I have missed something important and must go back and reread the passage at least two or three times.	Not at All	A little	Quite a Lot	A Lot	Very Much
24	I imagine catastrophic consequences as a result of absent-mindedness or minor errors which I make.	Not at All	A little	Quite a Lot	A Lot	Very Much
25	I think or worry at length about having hurt someone without knowing it.	Not at All	A little	Quite a Lot	A Lot	Very Much
26	When I hear about a disaster, I think it is somehow my fault.	Not at All	A little	Quite a Lot	A Lot	Very Much
27	I sometimes worry at length for no reason that I have hurt myself or have some disease.	Not at All	A little	Quite a Lot	A Lot	Very Much
28	I get upset and worried at the sight of knives, daggers, and other pointed objects.	Not at All	A little	Quite a Lot	A Lot	Very Much
29	When I hear about a suicide or a crime, I am upset for a long time and find it difficult to stop thinking about it.	Not at All	A little	Quite a Lot	A Lot	Very Much

30	I invent useless worries about germs and disease.	Not at All	A little	Quite a Lot	A Lot	Very Much
31	When I look down from a bridge or a very high window, I feel an impulse to throw myself into space.	Not at All	A little	Quite a Lot	A Lot	Very Much
32	When I see a train approaching, I sometimes think I could throw myself under its wheels.	Not at All	A little	Quite a Lot	A Lot	Very Much
33	At certain moments, I am tempted to tear off my clothes in public.	Not at All	A little	Quite a Lot	A Lot	Very Much
34	While driving, I sometimes feel an impulse to drive the car into someone or something.	Not at All	A little	Quite A Lot	A Lot	Very Much
35	Seeing weapons excites me and makes me think violent thoughts.	Not at All	A little	Quite a Lot	A Lot	Very Much
36	I sometimes feel the need to break or damage things for no reason.	Not at All	A little	Quite a Lot	A Lot	Very Much
37	I sometimes have an impulse to steal other people's belongings, even if they are of no use to me.	Not at All	A little	Quite aLot	A Lot	Very Much
38	I am sometimes almost irresistibly tempted to steal something from the supermarket.	Not at All	A little	Quite a Lot	A Lot	Very Much
39	I sometimes have an impulse to hurt defenseless children or animals.	Not at All	A little	Quite a Lot	A Lot	Very Much

Panic and Agoraphobia Scale (PAS)

Reference: **Bandelow B. Panic and Agoraphobia Scale (PAS). 1999. Seattle, WA, Hogrefe & Huber Publishers**

Rating Self-report or clinician-rated

Administration time 5–10 minutes

Main purpose To assess severity of panic disorder with or without agoraphobia

Population Adults and adolescents aged 15 and older

Commentary

The PAS is a 13-item measure of severity of illness in patients with panic disorder (with or without agoraphobia) over the past week. The instrument, available in both a self-report and clinician-rated format, contains 5 sub-scales: panic attacks, agoraphobic avoidance, anticipatory anxiety, disability and functional avoidance and health concerns. Although the PAS was originally developed to monitor the efficacy of pharmacological and psychotherapeutic interventions in clinical trials, it is appropriate for use in a variety of clinical or research environments.

Scoring

Items are rated on a 5-point scale ranging from 0–4 (anchors vary from item to item). The total score is computed by adding all item scores. The instrument provides a total score (range 0–52) as well as sub-scale scores, which are derived by calculating the mean of the appropriate items. The manual provides the following guidelines for interpreting scores derived from the clinician-rated version: 0–6 (in remission or borderline), 7–17 (mild), 18–28 (moderate), 29–39 (severe), ≥40 (very severe). Guidelines for the self-rated version are: 0–8 (in remission or borderline), 9–18 (mild), 19–28 (moderate), 29–39 (severe), ≥40 (very severe).

Versions

The PAS has been translated into: Afrikaans, Arabic, Danish, Dutch, French, German, Greek, Hebrew, Hungarian, Italian, Japanese, Polish, Portuguese, Russian, Serbocroat, Spanish, Swedish and Turkish. A computerized version is also available. See http://www.gwdg.de/~ukyp/pas.htm for further details.

Additional references

Bandelow B. Assessing the efficacy of treatments for panic disorder and agoraphobia. II. The Panic and Agoraphobia Scale. Int Clin Psychopharmacol 1995; 10(2):73–81.

Bandelow B, Broocks A, Pekrun G, George A, Meyer T, Pralle L, Bartmann U, Hillmer-Vogel U, Rüther E. The use of the Panic and Agoraphobia Scale (P & A) in a controlled clinical trial. Pharmacopsychiatry 2000; 33(5):174–81.

Address for correspondence

Hogrefe & Huber Publishers
P.O. Box 2487
Kirkland, WA 98033-2487, USA
Telephone: 1-425-820-1500
Email: hh@hhpub.com

Panic and Agoraphobia Scale

Patient:

Date:

Visit:

Rater:

Rate the past week!

A) panic attacks

A.1. Frequency
- ☐ 0 no panic attack in the past week
- ☐ 1 1 panic attack in the past week
- ☐ 2 2 or 3 panic attacks in the past week
- ☐ 3 4–6 panic attacks in the past week
- ☐ 4 more than 6 panic attacks in the past week

A.2. Severity
- ☐ 0 no panic attacks
- ☐ 1 attacks were usually very mild
- ☐ 2 attacks were usually moderate
- ☐ 3 attacks were usually severe
- ☐ 4 attacks were usually extremely severe

A.3. Average duration of panic attacks
- ☐ 0 no panic attacks
- ☐ 1 1 to 10 minutes
- ☐ 2 over 10 to 60 minutes
- ☐ 3 over 1 to 2 hours
- ☐ 4 over 2 hours and more

U. Were most of the attacks expected (occurring in feared situations) or unexpected (spontaneous)
- ☐ 9 no panic attacks
- ☐ 0 mostly unexpected
- ☐ 1 more unexpected than expected
- ☐ 2 some unexpected, some expected
- ☐ 3 more expected than unexpected
- ☐ 4 mostly expected

B) Agoraphobia, avoidance behaviour

B.1. Frequency of avoidance behaviour
- ☐ 0 no avoidance (or no agoraphobia)
- ☐ 1 infrequent avoidance of feared situations
- ☐ 2 occasional avoidance of feared situations
- ☐ 3 frequent avoidance of feared situations
- ☐ 4 very frequent avoidance of feared situations

B.2. Number of feared situations
How many situations are avoided or induce panic attacks or discomfort?
- ☐ 0 none (or no agoraphobia)
- ☐ 1 1 situation
- ☐ 2 2–3 situations
- ☐ 3 4–8 situations
- ☐ 4 occurred in very many different situations

B.3. Importance of avoided situations
How important are the avoided situations?
- ☐ 0 unimportant (or no agoraphobia)
- ☐ 1 not very important
- ☐ 2 moderately important
- ☐ 3 very important
- ☐ 4 extremely important

C) Anticipatory anxiety ('fear of fear')

C.1. Frequency of anticipatory anxiety
- ☐ 0 no fear of having a panic attack
- ☐ 1 infrequent fear of having a panic attack
- ☐ 2 sometimes fear of having a panic attack
- ☐ 3 frequent fear of having a panic attack
- ☐ 4 fear of having a panic attack all the time

C.2. How strong was this 'fear of fear'?
- ☐ 0 no
- ☐ 1 mild
- ☐ 2 moderate
- ☐ 3 marked
- ☐ 4 extreme

D) Disability

D.1. Disability in family relationships (partnership, children, etc.)
- ☐ 0 no
- ☐ 1 mild
- ☐ 2 moderate
- ☐ 3 marked
- ☐ 4 extreme

D.2. Disability in social relationships and leisure time (social events like cinema, etc.)
- ☐ 0 no
- ☐ 1 mild
- ☐ 2 moderate
- ☐ 3 marked
- ☐ 4 extreme

D.3. Disability in employment (or housework)
- ☐ 0 no
- ☐ 1 mild
- ☐ 2 moderate
- ☐ 3 marked
- ☐ 4 extreme

E) Worries about health

E.1. Worries about health damage
Patient was worried about suffering bodily damage due to the disorder
- ☐ 0 not true
- ☐ 1 hardly true
- ☐ 2 partly true
- ☐ 3 mostly true
- ☐ 4 definitely true

E.2. Assumption of organic disease
Patient thought that his anxiety symptoms are due to a somatic and not to a psychological disorder
- ☐ 0 not true, psychological disorder
- ☐ 1 hardly true
- ☐ 2 partly true
- ☐ 3 mostly true
- ☐ 4 definitely true, somatic disorder

☐ **Total score: Add all item scores except item U**

Panic and Agoraphobia Scale – patient questionnaire

Patient:

Date:

Visit:

This questionnaire is designed for people suffering from panic attacks and agoraphobia. Rate the severity of your symptoms in the **past week.**

Panic attacks are defined as the sudden outburst of anxiety, accompanied by some of the following symptoms:

- [ ] palpitations or pounding heart, or accelerated heart rate
- [ ] sweating
- [ ] trembling or shaking
- [ ] dry mouth
- [ ] difficulty in breathing
- [ ] feeling of choking
- [ ] chest pain or discomfort
- [ ] nausea or abdominal distress (e.g. churning in stomach)
- [ ] feeling dizzy, unsteady, faint, or light headed
- [ ] feelings that objects are unreal (like in a dream), or that the self is distant or 'not really here'
- [ ] fear of losing control, 'going crazy', or passing out
- [ ] fear of dying
- [ ] hot flushes or cold chills
- [ ] numbness or tingling sensations

Panic attacks develop suddenly and increase in intensity within about ten minutes

A.1. How frequently did you have panic attacks?
- [ ] 0 no panic attack in the past week
- [ ] 1 1 panic attack in the past week
- [ ] 2 2 or 3 panic attacks in the past week
- [ ] 3 4–6 panic attacks in the past week
- [ ] 4 more than 6 panic attacks in the past week

A.2. How severe were the panic attacks in the past week?
- [ ] 0 no panic attacks
- [ ] 1 attacks were usually mild
- [ ] 2 attacks were usually moderate
- [ ] 3 attacks were usually severe
- [ ] 4 attacks were usually extremely severe

A.3. How long did the panic attacks usually last?
- [ ] 0 no panic attacks
- [ ] 1 1 to 10 minutes
- [ ] 2 over 10 to 60 minutes
- [ ] 3 over 1 to 2 hours
- [ ] 4 over 2 hours and more

U. Were most of the attacks expected (occurring in feared situations) or unexpected (spontaneous)
- [ ] 9 no panic attacks
- [ ] 0 mostly unexpected
- [ ] 1 more unexpected than expected
- [ ] 2 some unexpected, some expected
- [ ] 3 more expected than unexpected
- [ ] 4 mostly expected

B.1. In the past week, did you avoid certain situations because you feared having a panic attack or a feeling of discomfort?
- [ ] 0 no avoidance (or my attacks don't occur in certain situations)
- [ ] 1 infrequent avoidance of feared situations
- [ ] 2 occasional avoidance of feared situations
- [ ] 3 frequent avoidance of feared situations
- [ ] 4 very frequent avoidance of feared situations

B.2. Please tick the situations you avoided or in which you developed panic attacks or a feeling of discomfort when you are not accompanied:
- [ ] Aeroplanes
- [ ] Subways (Underground)
- [ ] Buses, trains
- [ ] Ships
- [ ] Theatres, cinemas
- [ ] Supermarkets
- [ ] Standing in queues (lines)
- [ ] Auditoriums, stadiums
- [ ] Parties or social gatherings
- [ ] Crowds
- [ ] Restaurants
- [ ] Museums
- [ ] Lifts
- [ ] Enclosed spaces (e.g. tunnels)
- [ ] Classrooms, lecture theatres
- [ ] Driving or riding in a car (e.g. in a traffic jam)
- [ ] Large rooms (lobbies)
- [ ] Walking on the street
- [ ] Fields, wide streets, courtyards
- [ ] High places
- [ ] Crossing bridges
- [ ] Travelling away from home
- [ ] Staying at home alone

other situations:
- [ ] _____
- [ ] _____
- [ ] _____

B.3. How important were the avoided situations
How important are the avoided situations?
- [ ] 0 unimportant (or no agoraphobia)
- [ ] 1 not very important
- [ ] 2 moderately important
- [ ] 3 very important
- [ ] 4 extremely important

C.1. In the past week, did you suffer from the fear of having a panic attack (anticipatory anxiety or 'fear of being afraid')?
- [ ] 0 no anticipatory anxiety
- [ ] 1 infrequent fear of having a panic attack
- [ ] 2 sometimes fear of having a panic attack
- [ ] 3 frequent fear of having a panic attack
- [ ] 4 fear of having a panic attack all the time

C.2. How strong was this 'fear of fear'?
- [ ] 0 no
- [ ] 1 mild
- [ ] 2 moderate
- [ ] 3 marked
- [ ] 4 extreme

Panic and Agoraphobia Scale – patient questionnaire

D.1. In the past week, did your panic attacks or agoraphobia lead to restrictions (impairment) in your family relationships (partnership, children etc.)

- ☐ 0 no impairment
- ☐ 1 mild impairment
- ☐ 2 moderate impairment
- ☐ 3 marked impairment
- ☐ 4 extreme impairment

D.2. In the past week, did your panic attacks or agoraphobia lead to restrictions (impairment) in your social life and leisure activities (e.g. weren't you able to go to a cinema or to parties?)

- ☐ 0 no impairment
- ☐ 1 mild impairment
- ☐ 2 moderate impairment
- ☐ 3 marked impairment
- ☐ 4 extreme impairment

D.3. In the past week, did your panic attacks or agoraphobia lead to restrictions (impairment) in your work (or household) responsibilities?

- ☐ 0 no impairment
- ☐ 1 mild impairment
- ☐ 2 moderate impairment
- ☐ 3 marked impairment
- ☐ 4 extreme impairment

E.1. In the past week, did you worry about suffering harm from your anxiety symptoms (e.g. having a heart attack or collapsing and being injured?)

- ☐ 0 not true
- ☐ 1 hardly true
- ☐ 2 partly true
- ☐ 3 mostly true
- ☐ 4 definitely true

E.2. Did you sometimes think/believe that your doctor was wrong when he told you that your symptoms like pounding heart, dizziness, tingling sensations, shortness of breath, have a psychological cause? Did you believe that, in reality, a somatic (physical, bodily) cause lies behind these symptoms that hasn't been found yet?

- ☐ 0 not at all true (rather psychic disease)
- ☐ 1 hardly true
- ☐ 2 partly true
- ☐ 3 mostly true
- ☐ 4 definitely true (rather organic disease)

Panic Disorder Severity Scale (PDSS)

Reference: **Shear MK, Brown TA, Barlow DH, Money R, Sholomskas DE, Woods SW, Gorman JM, Papp LA. Multicenter collaborative panic disorder severity scale. Am J Psychiatry 1997; 154(11):1571–5**

Rating Clinician-rated

Administration time 10 minutes

Main purpose To assess severity of panic disorder

Population Adults

Commentary

The PDSS is a 7-item instrument to rate overall severity of DSM-IV panic disorder in patients who have already been diagnosed with the condition. Previous versions of the scale included the Cornell-Yale Panic Anxiety Scale (CY-PAS), and the Multicenter Panic-Anxiety Scale (MC-PAS). The instrument assesses symptoms over the past month, although alternative assessment periods may be used. The PDSS provides a number of indices, including frequency of panic attacks, distress during panic attacks, panic-focused anticipatory anxiety, avoidance of agoraphobic situations, avoidance of panic-related physical sensations, and impairment in social and occupational functioning. The scale represents a psychometrically sound method of assessing severity of panic disorder symptoms and treatment outcome.

Scoring

Items are scored on a 0 (none or not present) to 4 (extreme, pervasive, near-constant symptoms, disabling/incapacitating) scale, with a total score range of 0–28. The scale developers suggest that a cut-off score of 8 should be used if screening for diagnosis-level symptoms of panic disorder.

Versions

A self report version (the PDSS-SR) has recently been developed and the scale has been translated in Turkish.

Additional references

Barlow DH, Gorman JM, Shear MK, Woods SW. Cognitive-behavioral therapy, imipramine, or their combination for panic disorder: A randomized controlled trial. JAMA 2000; 283(19):2529–36.

Shear MK, Rucci P, Williams J, Frank E, Grochocinski V, Vander Bilt J, Houck P, Wang T. Reliability and validity of the Panic Disorder Severity Scale: replication and extension. J Psychiatr Res 2001; 35(5):293–6.

Houck PR, Spiegel DA, Shear MK, Rucci P. Reliability of the self-report version of the panic disorder severity scale. Depress Anxiety 2002; 15(4):183–5.

Address for correspondence

Dr. Katherine Shear
Anxiety Disorders Prevention Program
Western Psychiatric Institute and Clinic
University of Pittsburgh
3811 O'Hara Street
Pittsburgh, PA 15213-2593, USA
Telephone: 1-412-624-5500
Email: Shearmk@msx.upmc.edu

Panic Disorder Severity Scale

TIME PERIOD OF RATING   (Circle one):   one month
                                                  other (specify) _____

General Instructions for Raters

The goal is to obtain a measure of overall severity of DSM IV symptoms of panic disorder, with or without agoraphobia. Ratings are generally made for the past month, to allow for a stable estimation of panic frequency and severity. Users may choose a different time frame, but time frame should be consistent for all items.

Each item is rated from 0–4, where 0 = none or not present; 1 = mild, occasional symptoms, slight interference; 2 = moderate, frequent symptoms, some interference with functioning, but still manageable; 3 = severe, preoccupying symptoms, substantial interference in functioning, and 4 = extreme, pervasive near constant symptoms, disabling/incapacitating.

A suggested script is provided as a guide to questioning, but is not essential. Probes should be used freely to clarify ratings. As an overall caution, please note that this is not an observer administered self-rating scale. The patient is not asked to rate a symptom as 'mild, moderate or severe'. Rather the symptom is explored and rated by the interviewer. However, to clarify a boundary between two severity levels, it is appropriate to utilize the descriptors above. For example, the interviewer might ask the patient whether it is more accurate to describe a given symptom as occurring 'frequently, with definite interference but still manageable', or if it is 'preoccupying, with substantial interference'. Similarly, it might be appropriate to ask whether a symptom is 'preoccupying, with substantial interference', or 'pervasive, near constant, and incapacitating'.

In rating items 6 and 7, the interviewer should be alert to incosistencies. For example, sometimes a subject will describe a symptom from items 1–5 as causing substantial impairment in functioning, but then will report that overall panic disorder symptoms cause only mild or moderate work and social impairment. This should be pointed out and clarified.

There are some types of anxiety, common in panic disorder patients, but not rated by this instrument. Anticipatory anxiety about situations feared for reasons other than panic (e.g. related to a specific phobia or social phobia) is not considered panic-related anticipatory anxiety and is not rated by this instrument. Similarly, generalized anxiety is not rated by this instrument. The concerns of someone experiencing generalized anxiety are focused on the probability of adverse events in the future. Such worries often include serious health problems in oneself or a loved one, financial ruin, job loss, or other possible calamitous outcomes of daily life problems.

1. PANIC ATTACK FREQUENCY, INCLUDING LIMITED SYMPTOM EPISODES

Begin by explaining to the patient that we define a *Panic Attack* as a feeling of fear or apprehension that begins suddenly and builds rapidly in intensity, usually reaching a peak in less than 10 minutes. This feeling is associated with uncomfortable physical sensations like racing or pounding heart, shortness of breath, choking, dizziness, sweating, trembling. Often there are distressing, catastrophic thoughts such as fear of losing control, having a heart attack or dying. A full panic episode has at least four such symptoms. A *Limited Symptom Episode* (LSE) is similar to a full panic attack, but has fewer than 4 symptoms. Given these definitions, please tell me

Q: In the past month, how many full panic attacks did you experience, the kind with 4 or more symptoms? How about limited symptom episodes, the kind with less than 4 symptoms? On average, did you have more than one limited symptom episodes/day? *(Calculate weekly frequencies by dividing the total number of full panic attacks over the rating interval by the number of weeks in the rating interval.)*

0 = No panic or limited symptom episodes

1 = Mild, less than an average of one full panic a week, and no more than 1 limited symptom episode/day

2 = Moderate, one or two full panic attacks a week, and/or multiple limited symptom episodes/day

3 = Severe, more than 2 full attacks/week, but not more than 1/day on average

4 = Extreme, full panic attacks occur more than once a day, more days than not

2. DISTRESS DURING PANIC ATTACKS, INCLUDE LIMITED SYMPTOM EPISODES

Q: Over the past month, when you had panic or limited symptom attacks, how much distress did they cause you? I am asking you now about the distress you felt during the attack itself.

(This item rates the average degree of distress and discomfort the patient experienced during panic attacks experienced over the rating interval. Limited symptom episodes should be rated only if they caused more distress than full panic. be sure to distinguish between distress DURING panic and anticipatory fear that an attack will occur.)

Possible further probes: How upset or fearful did you feel during the attacks? Were you able to continue doing what you were doing when panic occurred? Did you lose your concentration? If you had to stop what you were doing, were you able to stay in the situation where the attack occurred or did you have to leave?

0 = No panic attacks or limited symptom episodes, or no distress during episodes

1 = Mild distress but able to continue activity with little or no interference

2 = Moderate distress, but still manageable, able to continue activity and/or maintain concentration, but does so with difficulty

3 = Severe, marked distress and interference, loses concentration and/or must stop activity, but able to remain in the room or situation

4 = Extreme, severe and disabling distress, must stop activity, will leave the room or situation if possible, otherwise remains, unable to concentrate, with extreme distress

3. SEVERITY OF ANTICIPATORY ANXIETY (panic-related fear, apprehension or worry)

Q: Over the past month, on average, how much did you worry, feel fearful or apprehensive about when your next panic would occur or about what panic attacks might mean about your physical or mental health? I am asking about times when you were not actually having a panic attack.

(Anticipatory anxiety can be related to the meaning of the attacks rather than to having an attack, so there can be considerable anxiety about having an attack even if the distress during the attacks was low. Remember that sometimes a patient does not worry about when the next attack will occur, but instead worries about the meaning of the attacks for his or her physical or mental health.)

Possible further probes: How intense was your anxiety? How often did you have these worries or fears? Did the anxiety get to the point where it interfered with your life? IF SO, how much did it interfere?

0 = No concern about panic

1 = Mild, there is occasional fear, worry or apprehension about panic

2 = Moderate, often worried, fearful or apprehensive, but has periods without anxiety. there is a noticeable modification of lifestyle, but anxiety is still manageable and overall functioning is not impaired

3 = Severe, preoccupied with fear, worry or apprehension about panic, substantial interference with concentration and/or ability to function effectively

4 = Extreme, near constant and disabling anxiety, unable to carry out important tasks because of fear, worry or apprehension about panic

4. AGORAPHOBIC FEAR/AVOIDANCE

Q: Over the past month, were there places where you felt afraid, or that you avoided, because you thought if you had a panic attack, it could be difficult to get help or to easily leave?
Possible further probes: Situations like using public transportation, driving in a car, being in a tunnel or on a bridge, going to the movies, to a mall or supermarket, or being in other crowded places? anywhere else? Were you afraid of being at home alone or completely alone in other places? How often did you experience fear of these situations? How intense was the fear? Did you avoid any of these situations? Did having a trusted companion with you make a difference? Were there things you would do with a companion that you would not do alone? How much did the fear and/or avoidance affect your life? Did you need to change your lifestyle to accommodate your fears?

0 = None, no fear or avoidance
1 = Mild, occasional fear and/or avoidance, but will usually confront or endure the situation. There is little or no modification of lifestyle
2 = Moderate, noticeable fear and/or avoidance, but still manageable, avoids feared situations but can confront with a companion. There is some modification of lifestyle, but overall functioning is not impaired
3 = Severe, extensive avoidance; substantial modification of lifestyle is required to accommodate phobia, making it difficult to manage usual activities
4 = Extreme pervasive disabling fear and/or avoidance. Extensive modification in lifestyle is required such that important tasks are not performed.

5. PANIC-RELATED SENSATION FEAR/AVOIDANCE

Q: Sometimes people with panic disorder experience physical sensations that may be reminiscent of panic and cause them to feel frightened or uncomfortable. Over the past month, did you avoid doing anything because you thought it might cause this kind of uncomfortable physical sensations?
Possible further probes: For example, things that made your heart beat rapidly, such as strenuous exercise or walking? playing sports? working in the garden? What about exciting sports events, frightening movies or having an argument? Sexual activity or orgasm? Did you fear or avoid sensations on your skin such as heat or tingling? Sensations of feeling dizzy or out of breath? Did you avoid any food, drink or other substance because it might bring on physical sensations, such as coffee or alcohol or medications like cold medication? How much did the avoidance of situations or activities like these affect your life? Did you need to change your lifestyle to accommodate your fears?

0 = no fear or avoidance of situations or activities that provoke distressing physical sensations
1 = Mild, occasional fear and/or avoidance, but usually will confront or endure with little distress activities and situations which provoke physical sensations. There is little modification of lifestyle.
2 = Moderate, noticeable avoidance, but still manageable; there is definite, but limited modification of lifestyle, such that overall functioning is not impaired
3 = Severe, extensive avoidance, causes substantial modification of lifestyle or interference in functioning

4 = Extreme pervasive and disabling avoidance. Extensive modification in lifestyle is required such that important tasks or activities are not performed

6. IMPAIRMENT/INTERFERENCE IN WORK FUNCTIONING DUE TO PANIC DISORDER

(Note to raters: This item focuses on work. If the person is not working, ask about school, and if not in school full time, ask about household responsibilities.)
Q: Over the past month, considering all the symptoms, the panic attacks, limited symptom episodes, anticipatory anxiety and phobic symptoms, how much did your panic disorder interfere with your ability to do your job (or your schoolwork, or carry out responsibilities at home?)
Possible further probes: Did the symptoms affect the quality of your work? Were you able to get things done as quickly and effectively as usual? Did you notice things you were not doing because of your anxiety, or things you couldn't do as well? Did you take short cuts or request assistance to get things done? Did anyone else notice a change in your performance? Was there a formal performance review or warning about work performance? Any comments from co-workers or from family members about your work?

0 = No impairment from panic disorder symptoms
1 = Mild, slight interference, feels job is harder to do but performance is still good
2 = Moderate, symptoms cause regular, definite interference but still manageable. Job performance has suffered but others would say work is still adequate
3 = Severe, causes substantial impairment in occupational performance, such that others have noticed, may be missing work or unable to perform at all on some days
4 = Extreme, incapacitating symptoms, unable to work (or go to school or carry out household responsibilities)

7. IMPAIRMENT/INTERFERENCE IN SOCIAL FUNCTIONING DUE TO PANIC DISORDER

Q: Over the past month, considering all the panic disorder symptoms together, how much did they interfere with your social life?
Possible further probes: Did you spend less time with family or other relatives than you used to? Did you spend less time with friends? Did you turn down opportunities to socialize because of panic disorder? Did you have restrictions about where or how long you would socialize because of panic disorder? Did the panic disorder symptoms affect your relationships with family members or friends?

0 = No impairment
1 = Mild, slight interference, feels quality of social behaviour is somewhat impaired but social functioning is still adequate
2 = Moderate, definite, interference with social life but still manageable. There is some decrease in frequency of social activities and/or quality of interpersonal interactions but still able to engage in most usual social activities
3 = Severe, causes substantial impairment in social performance. There is marked decrease in social activities, and/or marked difficulty interacting with others; can still force self to interact with others, but does not enjoy or function well in most social or interpersonal situations
4 = Extreme, disabling symptoms, rarely goes out or interacts with others, may have ended a relationship because of panic disorder

TOTAL SCORE (sum of items 1–7):

_____

American Journal of Psychiatry, vol. 154, pp. 1571–5, 1997. Copyright 1997, the American Psychiatric Association; http://ajp.psychiatryonline.org. Reprinted by permission.

Penn State Worry Questionnaire (PSWQ)

Reference: **Meyer TJ, Miller ML, Metzger RL, Borkovec TD. Development and validation of the Penn State Worry Questionnaire. Behav Res Ther 1990; 28(6):487–95**

Rating Self-report

Administration time 5 minutes

Main purpose To assess trait symptoms of pathological worry

Population Adults

Commentary

The PSWQ is a 16-item self-report measure designed to assess the frequency and severity of symptoms of worry as typified by patients diagnosed with generalized anxiety disorder. Factor analyses have generally indicated that the PSWQ assesses a unidimensional construct. The scale is able to differentiate between patients with generalized anxiety disorder and those with other anxiety disorders such as panic disorder, social phobia and obsessive-compulsive disorder (Brown et al., 1992). Although the scale is not appropriate for use a diagnostic instrument for generalized anxiety disorder, it may prove useful as a screening tool for pathological worry and is sensitive to change in response to treatment. The instrument is reproduced in full here and is in the public domain.

Scoring

Items are rated on a 1 (not at all typical) to 5 (very typical) scale, and the instrument has a total score range of 16–80 (note some items are reverse scored).

Versions

The Penn State Worry Questionnaire - Past Week (PSWQ-PW) assesses worry over the previous week as opposed to trait worry, and represents a more useful tool for assessing treatment effects. A scale for children is available (PSWQ-C), and the instrument has been translated into Chinese, Dutch, French, German, Greek, Italian, Spanish and Thai.

Additional references

Brown TA, Antony MM, Barlow DH. Psychometric properties of the Penn State Worry Questionnaire in a clinical anxiety disorders sample. Behav Res Ther 1992; 30(1):33–7.

Molina S, Borkovec TD. The Penn State Worry Questionnaire: Psychometric properties and associated characteristics. In G. Davey and F. Tallis (Eds.) Worrying: Perspectives on theory, assessment, and treatment, pp. 265–83. 1994. Sussex, England: Wiley & Sons.

Stober J, Bittencourt J. Weekly assessment of worry: an adaptation of the Penn State Worry Questionnaire for monitoring changes during treatment. Behav Res Ther 1998; 36(6):645–56.

Chelminski I, Zimmerman M. Pathological worry in depressed and anxious patients. J Anxiety Disord 2003; 17(5):533–46.

Address for correspondence

Dr. Thomas D. Borkovec
Department of Psychology
544 Moore Building
Penn State University
University Park, PA 16802, USA
Telephone: 1-814-863-1725
Email: tdb@psu.edu

Penn State Worry Questionnaire (PSWQ)

Enter the number that best describes how typical or characteristic each item is of you, putting the number next to the item.

1	2	3	4	5
Not at all typical		Somewhat typical		Very typical

___   1.   If I don't have enough time to do everything I don't worry about it.

___   2.   My worries overwhelm me.

___   3.   I don't tend to worry about things.

___   4.   Many situations make me worry.

___   5.   I know I shouldn't worry about things, but I just can't help it.

___   6.   When I am under pressure I worry a lot.

___   7.   I am always worrying about something.

___   8.   I find it easy to dismiss worrisome thoughts.

___   9.   As soon as I finish one task, I start to worry about everything else I have to do.

___   10.   I never worry about anything.

___   11.   When there is nothing more I can do about a concern, I don't worry about it any more.

___   12.   I've been a worrier all my life.

___   13.   I notice that I have been worrying about things.

___   14.   Once I start worrying, I can't stop.

___   15.   I worry all the time.

___   16.   I worry about projects until they are all done.

(Reverse-score items 1, 3, 8, 10, and 11, and then sum over 16 items.)

Reproduced from Meyer TJ, Miller ML, Metzger RL, Borkovec TD. Behav Res Ther 1990; 28(6):487–95.

Posttraumatic Stress Diagnostic Scale (PDS)

Reference: **Foa EB, Cashman LA, Jaycox L, Perry K. The validation of a self-report measure of posttraumatic stress disorder: The Posttraumatic Diagnostic Scale. Psychol Assess 1997; 4:445–51**

Rating Self-report

Administration time 10–15 minutes

Main purpose To assess DSM-IV diagnostic criteria and symptom severity of PTSD

Population Adults

Commentary

The PDS (a revised version of the PTSD Symptom Scale) is a 49-item self-report measure that yields both a diagnosis of PTSD and acts as a measure of symptom severity. The scale contains 4 sections. In the first section, the patient is required to indicate from a checklist of 12 items which traumatic events they have experienced or witnessed. In the second section, the patient selects the event that has bothered them the most in the past month and states whether they or someone else was injured in the event, whether they perceived a threat to their own or someone else's life, and if the event caused feeling of helplessness and terror. The third section of the questionnaire assesses the 17 symptoms of PTSD outlined in DSM-IV. Finally, the fourth part of the scale assesses the impact of PTSD symptoms upon important areas of functioning (e.g. occupational, family, leisure). The scale shows relatively sound psychometric properties in terms of reliability and validity, although it does demonstrate strong correlations with measures of depression and anxiety, such as the Beck Depression Inventory (see page 10) and the State-Trait Anxiety Scale (see page 109). The PDS may be used as a screening tool for PTSD and to monitor change in response to treatment, but should not be used in isolation to diagnose the disorder.

Scoring

In section 3 of the scale, items are rated on a 0 (not at all, or only one time) through to 3 (5 or more times a week/almost always) scale. Scoring provides a PTSD diagnosis (a diagnosis is confirmed if all 6 DSM-IV criteria are met), a symptom severity score, details of number of symptoms endorsed, specifiers (acute, chronic or with delayed onset), and an impairment in functioning score.

Versions

A computer-administered version is available.

Additional references

Foa EB. Posttraumatic Stress Diagnostic Scale: Manual. 1995. Minneapolis, MN, National Computer Systems.

Sheeran T, Zimmerman M. Screening for posttraumatic stress disorder in a general psychiatric outpatient setting. J Consult Clin Psychol 2002; 70(4):961–6.

Rosner R, Powell S, Butollo W. Posttraumatic Stress Disorder three years after the siege of Sarajevo. J Clin Psychol 2003; 59(1):41–55.

Address for correspondence

Pearson Assessments (formerly NCS Assessments)
Telephone: 1-800-627-7271, ext. 3225 or
1-952-681-3225
Fax: 1-800-632-9011 or 1-952-681-3299
Email: pearsonassessments@pearson.com
Website: www.pearsonassessments.com

Social Phobia and Anxiety Inventory (SPAI)

Reference: **Turner SM, Beidel DC, Dancu CV, Stanley MA. An empirically derived inventory to measure social fears and anxiety: The Social Phobia and Anxiety Inventory. Psychol Assess 1989; 1:35–40**

Rating Self-report

Administration time 20–30 minutes

Main purpose To assess symptoms of social phobia as defined by DSM-IV

Population Adults and adolescents

Commentary

The SPAI is a 45-item self-report measure of social phobia and social anxiety that contains 2 sub-scales, a 32-item social phobia scale, and a 13-item agoraphobia index. Within the social phobia sub-scale, 21 items measure degree of distress associated with a variety of social settings; the respondent is required to provide separate responses for 4 different audience groups (strangers, authority figures, the opposite sex, and people in general). The remaining social phobia items assess somatic and cognitive symptoms before or during social situations and avoidance or escape. The agoraphobia sub-scale assesses whether the patient's social problems are related to fear of having a panic attack, as opposed to fear of negative evaluation by others. The SPAI is able to distinguish between patients with social phobia and other anxiety disorders (e.g. panic disorder with or without agoraphobia) and between patients with anxiety and control subjects. Furthermore, it is sensitive to change in response to treatment (the SPAI has been used as an outcome measure in predominantly behavioural treatment studies for social phobia). The length of the instrument will, however, limit its usefulness in some clinical settings, as will its detailed and somewhat time-consuming scoring system.

Scoring

Items are scored on a 7-point scale ranging from 1 (never) through to 7 (always). Score ranges are 0–192 for the social phobia scale and 0–78 for the agoraphobia scale. Sub-scale scores are derived by summing the items in each sub-scale. The SPAI difference score (previously called the total score) is calculated by subtracting the agoraphobia sub-scale score from the social phobia sub-scale score, and represents a purer measure of social phobia. A score ≥39 on the agoraphobia sub-scale may indicate the presence of panic disorder.

Versions

A child version of the questionnaire (the SPAI-C) is available, and the scale has been translated into: French-Canadian, German, Icelandic, South American Portuguese, Spanish and Swedish. A computerized scoring version is also available.

Additional references

Beidel DC, Turner SM, Cooley MR. Assessing reliable and clinically significant change in social phobia: validity of the social phobia and anxiety inventory. Behav Res Ther 1993; 31(3):331–7.

Turner SM, Beidel DC, Dancu, CV. Social Phobia and Anxiety Inventory: Manual. 1996. Toronto, Canada, Multi-Health Systems Inc.

Peters L. Discriminant validity of the Social Phobia and Anxiety Inventory (SPAI), the Social Phobia Scale (SPS) and the Social Interaction Anxiety Scale (SIAS). Behav Res Ther 2000; 38(9):943–50.

Address for correspondence

Multi-Health Systems Inc.
P.O. Box 950
North Tonawanda, NY 14120–0950, USA
Telephone: 1-800-456-3003 in the US or
1-416-492-2627 international
Website: www.mhs.com

Social Phobia Inventory (SPIN)

Reference: **Connor KM, Davidson JR, Churchill LE, Sherwood A, Foa E, Weisler RH. Psychometric properties of the Social Phobia Inventory (SPIN). New self-rating scale. Br J Psychiatry 2000; 176:379–86**

Rating Self-report

Administration time 10 minutes

Main purpose To measure fear, avoidance and physiological symptoms associated with social phobia

Population Adults

Commentary

The SPIN is a recently developed 17-item self-report measure of symptoms associated with social phobia over the past week that focuses in particular on the core symptoms of fear, avoidance, and physiological arousal. Preliminary psychometric evaluation of the instrument has indicated that is has good test–retest reliability, internal consistency and convergent and divergent validity, and is sensitive to treatment effects. A useful 3-item Mini-SPIN (Connor et al., 2001) has also been developed as a screening tool for generalized social anxiety disorder.

Scoring

Items are coded on a 0 (not at all) to 4 (extremely) scale; a total score (range 0–68) can be calculated by summing the scale's fear, avoidance and physiological arousal sub-scales. A SPIN score of 19 has been shown to distinguish between patients with social phobia and control subjects.

Versions

The SPIN has been translated into a number of languages, including: Chinese, Dutch, Finnish, French, German, Japanese, Portuguese and Spanish.

Additional references

Connor KM, Kobak KA, Churchill LE, Katzelnick D, Davidson JR. Mini-SPIN: A brief screening assessment for generalized social anxiety disorder. Depress Anxiety 2001; 14(2):137–40.

Tharwani HM, Davidson JR. Symptomatic and functional assessment of social anxiety disorder in adults. Psychiatr Clin North Am 2001; 24(4):643–59.

Address for correspondence

Dr. Kathryn M. Connor
Box 3812
Duke University Medical Center
Durham, NC 27710, USA
Telephone: 1-919-684-5849
Email: kathryn.connor@duke.edu

Social Phobia Scale (SPS) and Social Interaction Anxiety Scale (SIAS)

Reference: **Mattick RP, Clarke JC. Development and validation of measures of social phobia scrutiny fear and social interaction anxiety. Behav Res Ther 1998; 36(4):455–70**

Rating Self-report

Administration time 5 minutes each

Main purpose The SPS was developed to assess fear of being observed by others during routine activities, whereas the SIAS measures fear of social interaction.

Population Adults

Commentary

The SPS and SIAS are companion 20-item self-report measures, designed to respectively assess fear of being scrutinized when undertaking routine activities, and fear of social interaction more broadly. In common use, these scales are typically administered together and treated as sub-scales of a larger measure. Both instruments demonstrated good internal consistency and test–retest reliability in the original Mattick et al. study (1998). They also discriminated between patients with social phobia, agoraphobia and simple phobia, and between social phobia and control subjects, and are sensitive to treatment effects. Exploratory factor analysis (Safren et al., 1998) yielded 3 factors (interaction anxiety, anxiety about being observed by others, and fear that others will notice anxiety symptoms), although these all loaded on a higher-order factor of social anxiety.

Scoring

Items are rated on a 5-point scale from 0 (not at all characteristic or true of me) through to 4 (extremely characteristic or true of me). Both instruments are scored by summing all items (note some items in the SIAS are reverse-scored).

Versions

Both scales have been translated into numerous languages.

Additional references

Ries BJ, McNeil DW, Boone ML, Turk CL, Carter LE, Heimberg RG. Assessment of contemporary social phobia verbal report instruments. Behav Res Ther 1998; 36(10):983–94.

Safren SA, Turk CL, Heimberg RG. Factor structure of the Social Interaction Anxiety Scale and the Social Phobia Scale. Behav Res Ther 1998; 36(4):443–53.

Address for correspondence

Professor Richard P. Mattick
National Drug and Alcohol Research Centre
University of New South Wales
Randwick, NSW 2052, Australia
Telephone: 61 2 9398 9333
Email: r.mattick@unsw.edu.au

Social Interaction Anxiety Scale (SIAS)

For each question, please circle a number to indicate the degree to which you feel the statement is characteristic or true of you. The rating scale is as follows:

0 = Not at all characteristic or true of me
1 = Slightly characteristic or true of me
2 = Moderately characteristic or true of me

3 = Very characteristic or true of me
4 = Extremely characteristic or true of me

	Not at all	Slightly	Moderately	Very	Extremely
1. I get nervous if I have to speak with someone in authority (teacher, boss, etc.)	0	1	2	3	4
2. I have difficulty making eye-contact with others	0	1	2	3	4
3. I become tense if I have to talk about myself or my feelings	0	1	2	3	4
4. I find difficulty mixing comfortably with the people I work with	0	1	2	3	4
5. I find it easy to make friends my own age	0	1	2	3	4
6. I tense-up if I meet an acquaintance in the street	0	1	2	3	4
7. When mixing socially, I am uncomfortable	0	1	2	3	4
8. I feel tense if I am alone with just one person	0	1	2	3	4
9. I am at ease meeting people at parties, etc.	0	1	2	3	4
10. I have difficulty talking with other people	0	1	2	3	4
11. I find it easy to think of things to talk about	0	1	2	3	4
12. I worry about expressing myself in case I appear awkward	0	1	2	3	4
13. I find it difficult to disagree with another's point of view	0	1	2	3	4
14. I have difficulty talking to an attractive person of the opposite sex	0	1	2	3	4
15. I find myself worrying that I won't know what to say in social situations	0	1	2	3	4
16. I am nervous mixing with people I don't know very well	0	1	2	3	4
17. I feel I'll say something embarrassing when talking	0	1	2	3	4
18. When mixing in a group, I find myself worrying I will be ignored	0	1	2	3	4
19. I am tense mixing in a group	0	1	2	3	4
20. I am unsure whether to greet someone I know only slightly	0	1	2	3	4

Reproduced from Mattick RP, Clarke JC. Behav Res Ther 1998; 36(4):455–70 with permission from Elsevier.

Social Phobia Scale (SPS)

For each question, please circle a number to indicate the degree to which you feel the statement is characteristic or true of you. The rating scale is as follows:

0 = Not at all characteristic or true of me
1 = Slightly characteristic or true of me
2 = Moderately characteristic or true of me

3 = Very characteristic or true of me
4 = Extremely characteristic or true of me

	Not at all	Slightly	Moderately	Very	Extremely
1. I become anxious if I have to write in front of other people	0	1	2	3	4
2. I become self-conscious when using public toilets	0	1	2	3	4
3. I can suddenly become aware of my own voice of others listening to me	0	1	2	3	4
4. I get nervous that people are staring at me as I walk down the street	0	1	2	3	4
5. I fear I may blush when I am with others	0	1	2	3	4
6. I feel self-conscious if I have to enter a room where others are already seated	0	1	2	3	4
7. I worry about shaking or trembling when I'm watched by other people	0	1	2	3	4
8. I would get tense if I had to sit facing other people on a bus or a train	0	1	2	3	4
9. I get panicky that others might see me faint or be sick or ill	0	1	2	3	4
10. I would find it difficult to drink something if in a group of people	0	1	2	3	4
11. It would make me feel self-conscious to eat in front of a stranger at a restaurant	0	1	2	3	4
12. I am worried people will think my behaviour odd	0	1	2	3	4
13. I would get tense if I had to carry a tray across a crowded cafeteria	0	1	2	3	4
14. I worry I'll lose control of myself in front of other people	0	1	2	3	4
15. I worry I might do something to attract the attention of other people	0	1	2	3	4
16. When in an elevator, I am tense if people look at me	0	1	2	3	4
17. I can feel conspicuous standing in a line	0	1	2	3	4
18. I can get tense when I speak in front of other people	0	1	2	3	4
19. I worry my head will shake or nod in front of others	0	1	2	3	4
20. I feel awkward and tense if I know people are watching me	0	1	2	3	4

Reproduced from Mattick RP, Clarke JC. Behav Res Ther 1998; 36(4):455–70 with permission from Elsevier.

State-Trait Anxiety Inventory (Form Y) (STAI)

Reference: **Spielberger CD, Gorusch RL, Lushene RE. Manual for the State-Trait Anxiety Inventory. 1970. Palo Alto, CA, Consulting Psychologists Press**

Rating Self-report

Administration time 20 minutes

Main purpose To assess state and trait levels of anxiety

Population Adults, adolescents and children

Commentary

The STAI Form Y is one of the more widely used self-report scales for the evaluation of anxiety in medical and, to a lesser extent, psychiatric patients (Form Y is a revised version of the original Form X). The instrument includes separate measures of state and trait anxiety – respondents are asked to indicate on two 20-item scales how they are feeling 'right now, at this moment' (state version) and how they 'generally' feel (trait version). The STAI shows good correlations with other measures of anxiety such as the Beck Anxiety Inventory (see page 68) and the Fear Questionnaire (see page 79). Due to its longevity and ease of acquisition and use, the STAI has been widely used in a variety of research studies and clinical settings. A 6-item short-form is also available.

Scoring

Items are scored on a 4-point scale; a total score (range 20–80) for each 20-item scale is calculated by summing the items (note some are reverse-scored). The scale developers suggest that scores in the range of 20–39 indicate low anxiety, 40–59, moderate anxiety, and 60–80, high anxiety.

Versions

The STAI has been translated into more than 40 languages including: Arabic, Chinese, Dutch, French, German, Hindi, Italian, Japanese, Korean, Polish, Portuguese, Russian and Spanish. A child version (the STAIC) and a Children–Parent Report-Trait Version (STAIC-P-T) have been developed. A computerized version is available from Multi-Health Systems Inc. (www.mhs.com).

Additional references

Spielberger CD. State-trait Anxiety Inventory: A Comprehensive Bibliography. 1989 Second Ed. Consultant Psychologists Press. Palo Alto, CA.

Marteau TM, Bekker H. The development of a six-item short-form of the state scale of the Spielberger State-Trait Anxiety Inventory (STAI). Br J Clin Psychol 1992; 31(3):301–6.

Kennedy BL, Schwab JJ, Morris RL, Beldia G. Assessment of state and trait anxiety in subjects with anxiety and depressive disorders. Psychiatr Q 2001; 72(3):263–76.

Address for correspondence

Mind Garden, Inc.
1690 Woodside Road, Suite 202
Redwood City, CA 94061, USA
Telephone: 1-650-261-3500
Email: info@mindgarden.com
Website: www.mindgarden.com

State-Trait Anxiety Inventory (Form Y) – sample items

INSTRUCTIONS

Statements that people use to describe themselves are given below. For each statement, please **circle** the appropriate number to indicate how you **generally** feel.

	Almost never	Sometimes	Often	Almost always
• I feel nervous and restless	1	2	3	4
• I feel like a failure	1	2	3	4
• I have disturbing thoughts	1	2	3	4
• I feel inadequate	1	2	3	4
• I am a steady person	1	2	3	4

Yale-Brown Obsessive Compulsive Scale (Y-BOCS)

References: **Goodman WK, Price LH, Rasmussen SA, Mazure C, Fleischmann RL, Hill CL, Heninger GR, Charney DS. The Yale-Brown Obsessive Compulsive Scale. I. Development, use, and reliability. Arch Gen Psychiatry 1989; 46(11):1006–11.**

Goodman WK, Price LH, Rasmussen SA, Mazure C, Delgado P, Heninger GR, Charney DS. The Yale-Brown Obsessive Compulsive Scale. II. Validity. Arch Gen Psychiatry 1989; 46(11):1012–16

Rating Clinician-administered

Administration time 20–30 minutes (will decrease with repeat administrations)

Main purpose To measure severity of obsessive-compulsive symptoms

Population Adults

Commentary

The Y-BOCS is the gold standard of clinician-administered scales for the assessment of obsessive-compulsive symptoms. A 64-item checklist to identify the content of obsessive-compulsive symptoms is administered prior to the administration of the actual Y-BOCS; the patient is then asked to focus on the 3 symptoms that cause the most distress during the semi-structured interview. The scale itself contains 2 sub-scales, one assessing obsessions, the other compulsions. The Y-BOCS is the best-available assessment tool for evaluating treatment outcome in patients with obsessive-compulsive disorder and symptom severity. It should not, however, be used in isolation as a diagnostic measure (it does not directly assess DSM-IV criteria). Although it is appropriate for use as a screening instrument, the scale's length may prohibit its use as such in some clinical settings.

Scoring

Both the obsessions and compulsions sub-scales are rated on a 5-point scale ranging from 0 (no symptoms) through to 4 (extreme symptoms). Detailed anchor points and probes are provided. Scores are summed to provide a total score (range 0–40) and sub-scale scores for obsessions (range 0–20) and compulsions (range 0–20). In clinical trials, a total score of ≥16 is typically used as an inclusion criteria.

Versions

A number of alternative versions of the scale have been developed, including a 10-item shopping version (YBOCS-SV), a 12-item scale for Body Dysmorphic Disorder (BDD-YBOCS), a 10-item version for heavy drinkers (Y-BOCS-hd), a 10-item trichotillomania scale (YBOCS-TM), and an interview for children (CY-BOCS). The instrument can also be administered in a self-report format (administration time approximately 10–15 minutes) either by paper-and-pencil, or via computer. The Y-BOCS has been translated into approximately 25 languages. A clinical interactive voice response (IVR) version is available from Healthcare Technology Systems, Inc.

Additional references

Kim SW, Dysken MW, Kuskowski M. The Yale-Brown Obsessive-Compulsive Scale: a reliability and validity study. Psychiatry Res 1990; 34(1):99–106.

Steketee G, Frost R, Bogart K. The Yale-Brown Obsessive Compulsive Scale: interview versus self-report. Behav Res Ther 1996; 34(8):675–84.

Address for correspondence

Dr. Wayne K. Goodman
Department of Psychiatry
University of Florida College of Medicine
PO Box 100256 Gainesville, FL 32610, USA
Telephone: 1-352-392-3681
Email: wkgood@psychiatry.ufl.edu

Yale-Brown Obsessive Compulsive Scale (Y-BOCS)

In this document: DSM-IV definition of OCD and Y-BOCS Evaluation Form

Diagnostic Criteria (DSM-IV 300.3 OCD)

A. The Person Exhibits Either Obsessions or Compulsions

Obsessions are indicated by the following:

- The person has recurrent and persistent thoughts, impulses, or images that are experienced, at some time during the disturbance, as intrusive and inappropriate and that cause marked anxiety or distress
- The thoughts, impulses, or images are not simply excessive worries about real-life problems
- The person attempts to ignore or suppress such thoughts, impulses, or images or to neutralize them with some other thought or action
- The person recognizes that the obsessional thoughts, impulses, or images are a product of his or her own mind (not imposed from without as in thought insertion)

Compulsions are indicated by the following:

- The person has repetitive behaviors (e.g., hand washing, ordering, checking) or mental acts (e.g., praying, counting, repeating words silently) that the person feels driven to perform in response to an obsession or according to rules that must be applied rigidly
- The behaviors or mental acts are aimed at preventing some dreaded event or situation; however, these behaviors or mental acts either are not connected in a realistic way with what they are designed to neutralize or prevent or are clearly excessive.

B. At some point during the course of the disorder, the person has recognized that the obsessions or compulsions are excessive or unreasonable. (Note: this does not apply to children.)

C. The obsessions or compulsions cause marked distress, are time consuming (take more than 1 hour a day), or significantly interfere with the person's normal routine, occupational/academic functioning, or usual social activities or relationships.

D. If another axis I disorder is present, the content of the obsessions or compulsions is not restricted to it (e.g., preoccupation with drugs in the presence of a substance abuse disorder).

E. The disturbance is not due to the direct physiologic effects of a substance (e.g., drug abuse, a medication) or a general medical condition.

Severity Ratings

Instructions: Check appropriate score. Choose only one number per item. Scores should reflect the composite effect of all obsessive compulsive symptoms. Rate the average occurrence of each item during the prior week up to and including now.

Obsession Rating Scale

1. Time spent on obsession
   - 0   0 hrs/day
   - 1   0–1 hrs/day
   - 2   1–3 hrs/day
   - 3   3–8 hrs/day
   - 4   8+ hrs/day
2. Interference from obsessions
   - 0   None
   - 1   Mild
   - 2   Definite but manageable
   - 3   Substantial impairment
   - 4   Incapacitating
3. Distress from obsessions
   - 0   None
   - 1   Little
   - 2   Moderate but manageable
   - 3   Severe
   - 4   Near constant, disabling
4. Resistance to obsessions
   - 0   Always resists
   - 1   Much resistance
   - 2   Some resistance
   - 3   Often yields
   - 4   Completely yields
5. Control over obsessions
   - 0   Complete control
   - 1   Much control
   - 2   Some control
   - 3   Little control
   - 4   No control

Compulsion Rating Scale

1. Time spent on compulsions
   - 0   0 hrs/day
   - 1   0–1 hrs/day
   - 2   1–3 hrs/day
   - 3   3–8 hrs/day
   - 4   8+ hrs/day
2. Interference from compulsions
   - 0   None
   - 1   Mild
   - 2   Definite but manageable
   - 3   Substantial impairment
   - 4   Incapacitating
3. Distress from compulsions
   - 0   None
   - 1   Little
   - 2   Moderate but manageable
   - 3   Severe
   - 4   Near constant, disabling
4. Resistance to compulsions
   - 0   Always resists
   - 1   Much resistance
   - 2   Some resistance
   - 3   Often yields
   - 4   Completely yields
5. Control over compulsions
   - 0   Complete control
   - 1   Much control
   - 2   Some control
   - 3   Little control
   - 4   No control

continued overleaf

Name _____   Date _____

Check all that apply, but clearly mark the principal symptoms with a 'p'.
(Rater must ascertain whether reported behaviours are bona fide symptoms of OCD, and not symptoms of another disorder such as simple phobia or hypochondrias. Items marked * may or may not be OCD phenomena.)

Current	Past	
		Aggressive obsessions
_____	_____	Fear might harm self
_____	_____	Fear might harm others
_____	_____	Violent or horrific images
_____	_____	Fear of blurting out obscenities or insults
_____	_____	Fear of doing something else embarrassing*
_____	_____	Fear will act on unwanted impulses (e.g., to stab friend)
_____	_____	Fear will steal things
_____	_____	Fear will harm others because not careful enough (e.g. hit/run MVA)
_____	_____	Fear will be responsible for something else terrible happening (e.g., fire, burglary)
_____	_____	Other
		Contamination obsessions
_____	_____	Concerns or disgust with bodily waste or secretions (e.g., urine, feces, saliva)
_____	_____	Concern with dirt or germs
_____	_____	Excessive concern with environmental contaminants (e.g. asbestos, radiation, toxic waste)
_____	_____	Excessive concern with household items (e.g., cleansers, solvents)
_____	_____	Excessive concern with animals (e.g. insects)
_____	_____	Bothered by sticky substances or residues
_____	_____	Concerned will get ill because of contaminant
_____	_____	Concerned will get others ill by spreading contaminant (aggressive)
_____	_____	No concern with consequences of contamination other than how it might feel
_____	_____	Other
		Sexual obsessions
_____	_____	Forbidden or perverse sexual thoughts, images, or impulses
_____	_____	Content involves children or incest
_____	_____	Content involves homosexuality*
_____	_____	Sexual behavior toward others (aggressive)*
_____	_____	Other
		Hoarding/saving obsessions
_____	_____	(distinguish from hobbies and concern with objects of monetary or sentimental value)
		Religious obsessions (scrupulosity)
_____	_____	Concerned with sacrilege and blasphemy
_____	_____	Excess concern with right/wrong, morality
_____	_____	Other
		Obsession with need for symmetry or exactness
_____	_____	Accompanied by magical thinking (e.g., concerned that mother will have accident unless things are in the right place)
_____	_____	Not accompanied by magical thinking
		Miscellaneous obsessions
_____	_____	Need to know or remember
_____	_____	Fear of saying certain things
_____	_____	Fear of not saying just the right thing
_____	_____	Fear of losing things
_____	_____	Intrusive (nonviolent) images
_____	_____	Intrusive nonsense sounds, words, or music
_____	_____	Bothered by certain sounds/noises*
_____	_____	Lucky/unlucky numbers
_____	_____	Colors with special significance
_____	_____	Superstitious fears
_____	_____	Other

Somatic obsessions

——— ——— Concern with illness or disease*
——— ——— Excessive concern with body part or aspect of appearance (e.g., dysmorphophobia)*
——— ——— Other

Cleaning/washing compulsions

——— ——— Excessive or ritualized handwashing
——— ——— Excessive or ritualized showering, bathing, toothbrushing, grooming or toilet routine
——— ——— Involves cleaning of household items or other inanimate objects
——— ——— Other measures to prevent or remove contact with contaminants
——— ——— Other

Checking compulsions

——— ——— Checking locks, stove, appliances, etc.
——— ——— Checking that did not/will not harm others
——— ——— Checking that did not/will not harm self
——— ——— Checking that nothing terrible did/will happen
——— ——— Checking that did not make mistake
——— ——— Checking tied to somatic obsessions
——— ——— Other

Repeating rituals

——— ——— Rereading or rewriting
——— ——— Need to repeat routine activities (e.g., in/out door, up/down from chair)
——— ——— Other

——— ——— **Counting compulsions**

——— ——— **Ordering/arranging compulsions**

Hoarding/collecting compulsions

——— ——— (distinguish from hobbies and concern with objects of monetary or sentimental value, e.g., carefully reads junk mail, piles up old newspapers, sorts through garbage, collects useless objects)

Miscellaneous compulsions

——— ——— Mental rituals (other than checking/counting)
——— ——— Excessive listmaking
——— ——— Need to tell, ask, or confess
——— ——— Need to touch, tap, or rub*
——— ——— Rituals involving blinking or staring*
——— ——— Measures (not checking) to prevent
——— ——— harm to self _____ harm to others _____ terrible consequences _____
——— ——— Ritualized eating behaviors*
——— ——— Superstitious behaviors
——— ——— Trichotillomania*
——— ——— Other self-damaging or self-mutilating behaviors*
——— ——— Other

Zung Self-Rating Anxiety Scale (SAS)

Reference: **Zung WW. A rating instrument for anxiety disorders. Psychosomatics 1971; 12(6):371–9**

Rating Self-report

Administration time 5 minutes

Main purpose To measure symptoms of anxiety

Population Adults

Commentary

The SAS (also know as the Zung SAS or the SRAS) is a 20-item self-report measure developed to assess symptoms of anxiety as described in DSM-II. The instrument primarily evaluates somatic symptoms of anxiety. The SAS has in the past been used in a variety of psychological and pharmacological treatment studies as an outcome measure, but has been used less of late.

Scoring

Items are scored on a 4-point scale ranging from 1 (none or a little of the time) through to 4 (most or all of the time), with some reverse scoring. A mean index score is derived by dividing the raw score by the maximum possible score of 80, and then multiplying by 100.

Versions

The SAS has been translated into Chinese, Dutch, Finnish, French, German, Italian, Japanese, Norwegian, Russian, Portuguese and Spanish.

Additional reference

Zung WW, Magruder-Habib K, Velez R, Alling W. The comorbidity of anxiety and depression in general medical patients: a longitudinal study. J Clin Psychiatry 1990; 51 Suppl:77–80.

Address for correspondence

None available

Zung Self-rating Anxiety Scale (SAS)

Purpose: To use the Self-rating Anxiety Scale (SAS) to assess the level of anxiety being experienced by the patient

Please read the following statements. Enter an 'x' in the appropriate column best describing your personal feelings (give only 1 answer per row)

	None or a little of the time	Some of the time	A good part of the time	Most or all of the time
I feel more nervous and anxious than usual.				
I feel afraid for no reason at all.				
I get upset easily or feel panicky.				
I feel like I'm falling apart and going to pieces.				
I feel that everything is all right and nothing bad will happen.				
My arms and legs shake and tremble.				
I am bothered by headaches, neck and back pain.				
I feel weak and get tired easily.				
I feel calm and can sit still easily.				
I can feel my heart beating fast.				
I am bothered by dizzy spells.				
I have fainting spells or feel like it.				
I can breathe in and out easily.				
I get feelings of numbness and tingling in my fingers and toes.				
I am bothered by stomach aches or indigestion.				
I have to empty my bladder often.				
My hands are usually dry and warm.				
My face gets hot and blushes.				
I fall asleep easily and get a good night's rest.				
I have nightmares.				

Reproduced from Zung WW. Psychosomatics 1971; 12(6):371–9.

Chapter 4

Related symptoms, side-effects, functioning and quality of life

There are various symptom criteria for depressive and anxiety disorders, but there are also many symptoms that are commonly associated with, but not specific to, these conditions. In particular, physical symptoms such as fatigue, dizziness, stomach and chest pain, muscle aches, and headaches are often experienced by people with depression or anxiety. One study by Simon and colleagues found that 69% of patients with major depression in primary care presented with *only* physical symptoms as the initial problem. Painful somatic conditions and symptoms are particularly prevalent in geriatric depression and anxiety.

Sexual dysfunction, including decreased libido, erectile and orgasm difficulties, is also very common in depression and anxiety. These symptoms are often masked because patients find it difficult to disclose such symptoms and many clinicians are uncomfortable discussing the topic. People experiencing depression also have negative cognitions, pessimism, hopelessness, low self-confidence and self-esteem. Cognitive distortions may include catastrophizing, magnifying negative events and discounting positive ones. Hopelessness remains one of the most reliable predictors of acute suicidal ideation and intent. Evidence-based psychotherapies can target either the cognitive distortions and dysfunctional behaviours or the disturbed interpersonal relationships in people with depression and/or anxiety.

Medication treatment is effective for mood and anxiety disorders, but all medications have the potential for side effects. Many of the side effects of newer medications mimic symptoms of depression, such as gastrointestinal disturbances, headaches, insomnia or somnolence, fatigue, and sexual dysfunction. Adjunctive treatments such as typical and atypical antipsychotic medications may have other adverse effects such as extrapyramidal side effects. One of the top reasons given for medication non-adherence is troublesome side effects.

The objective of treatment for mood and anxiety disorders is recovery, which is defined as full remission of symptoms *and* return to premorbid psychosocial functioning. Psychosocial functioning can be measured in a number of domains relating to work, play and relationships. There is increasing interest in quality of life (QoL) as an outcome measure for treatment. Quality of life is a broad concept, but basically refers to an individual's well-being in a variety of life domains, such as occupational, emotional, social and physical functioning. It is also a highly individual and personal concept; what may be essential in determining one person's QoL may be unimportant to another. Factors such as these make QoL challenging to measure properly, but it nevertheless remains an important aspect of patient well-being to capture. QoL assessment scales allow the patient to assess the impact of treatment interventions upon areas of their lives that may be of particular importance to them, such as their ability to enjoy their chosen leisure activities, or the quality of their intimate relationships. Some evidence has suggested that improvement in psychosocial functioning and QoL also occurs more slowly than improvement in symptoms. Traditional symptomatic assessment scales miss this valuable 'fine grain' information, which can greatly enrich the clinical picture and help the clinician better assess the effects of treatment upon broader areas of functioning.

Abnormal Involuntary Movement Scale (AIMS)

Reference: **Guy W. ECDEU Assessment Manual for Psychopharmacology: Revised (DHEW publication number ADM 76-338). Rockville, MD, US Department of Health, Education and Welfare, Public Health Service, Alcohol, Drug Abuse and Mental Health Administration, NIMH Psychopharmacology Research Branch, Division of Extramural Research Programs, 1976: 534–7**

Rating Clinician-rated

Administration time 5 minutes

Main purpose To assess level of dyskinesias in patients taking neuroleptic medications

Population Adults

Commentary

The AIMS is a 12-item clinician-rated scale to assess severity of dyskinesias (specifically, orofacial movements and extremity and truncal movements) in patients taking neuroleptic medications. Additional items assess the overall severity, incapacitation, and the patient's level of awareness of the movements, and distress associated with them. The AIMS has been used extensively to assess tardive dyskinesia in clinical trials of antipsychotic medications. Due to its simple design and short assessment time, the AIMS can easily be integrated into a routine clinical evaluation by the clinician or another trained rater.

Scoring

Items are scored on a 0 (none) to 4 (severe) basis; the scale provides a total score (items 1 through 7) or item 8 can be used in isolation as an indication of overall severity of symptoms.

Versions

Modified versions of the AIMS scale have been developed.

Additional references

Lane RD, Glazer WM, Hansen TE, Berman WH, Kramer SI. Assessment of tardive dyskinesia using the Abnormal Involuntary Movement Scale. J Nerv Ment Dis 1985; 173(6):353–7.

Munetz MR, Benjamin S. How to examine patients using the Abnormal Involuntary Movement Scale. Hosp Community Psychiatry 1988; 39(11):1172–7.

Address for correspondence

Not applicable – the scale is in the public domain.

Abnormal Involuntary Movement Scale (AIMS)

Instructions
There are two parallel procedures, the <u>examination procedure</u>, which tells the patient what to do, and the <u>scoring procedure</u>, which tells the clinician how to rate what he or she observes.

Examination Procedure
Either before or after completing the examination procedure, observe the patient unobtrusively at rest (e.g., in the waiting room).

The chair to be used in this examination should be a hard, firm one without arms.

1. Ask the patient whether there is anything in his or her mouth (such as gum or candy) and, if so, to remove it.
2. Ask about the 'current' condition of the patient's teeth. Ask if he or she wears dentures. Ask whether teeth or dentures bother the patient 'now'.
3. Ask whether the patient notices any movements in his or her mouth, face, hands, or feet. If yes, ask the patient to describe them and to indicate to what extent they 'currently' bother the patient or interfere with activities.
4. Have the patient sit in the chair with hands on knees, legs slightly apart, and feet flat on floor. (Look at the entire body for movements while the patient is in this position.)
5. Ask the patient to sit with hands hanging unsupported – if male, between his legs, if female and wearing a dress, hanging over her knees. (Observe hands and other body areas.)
6. Ask the patient to open his or her mouth. (Observe the tongue at rest within the mouth.) Do this twice.
7. Ask the patient to protrude his or her tongue. (Observe abnormalities of tongue movement.) Do this twice.
8. Ask the patient to tap his or her thumb with each finger as rapidly as possible for 10 to 15 seconds, first with right hand, then with left hand. (Observe facial and leg movements.) [±activated]
9. Flex and extend the patient's left and right arms, one at a time.
10. Ask the patient to stand up. (Observe the patient in profile. Observe all body areas again, hips included.)
11. Ask the patient to extend both arms out in front, palms down. (Observe trunk, legs, and mouth.) [activated]
12. Have the patient walk a few paces, turn, and walk back to the chair. (Observe hands and gait.) Do this twice. [activated]

Scoring Procedure
Complete the examination procedure before making ratings.

For the movement ratings (the first three categories below), rate the highest severity observed. 0 = none, 1 = minimal (may be extreme normal), 2 = mild, 3 = moderate, and 4 = severe. According to the <u>original</u> AIMS instructions, one point is subtracted if movements are seen **only on activation**, but not all investigators follow that convention.

Facial and Oral Movements
1. Muscles of facial expression,
   e.g., movements of forehead, eyebrows, periorbital area, cheeks. Include frowning, blinking, grimacing of upper face.
   0 1 2 3 4
2. Lips and perioral area,
   e.g., puckering, pouting, smacking.
   0 1 2 3 4
3. Jaw,
   e.g., biting, clenching, chewing, mouth opening, lateral movement.
   0 1 2 3 4
4. Tongue.
   Rate only increase in movement both in and out of mouth, **not** inability to sustain movement.
   0 1 2 3 4

Extremity Movements
5. Upper (arms, wrists, hands, fingers).
   Include movements that are choreic (rapid, objectively purposeless, irregular, spontaneous) or athetoid (slow, irregular, complex, serpentine). Do **not** include tremor (repetitive, regular, rhythmic movements).
   0 1 2 3 4
6. Lower (legs, knees, ankles, toes),
   e.g., lateral knee movement, foot tapping, heel dropping, foot squirming, inversion and eversion of foot.
   0 1 2 3 4

Trunk Movements
7. Neck, shoulders, hips,
   e.g., rocking, twisting, squirming, pelvic gyrations. Include diaphragmatic movements.
   0 1 2 3 4

Global Judgments
8. Severity of abnormal movements.
   0 1 2 3 4
   based on the highest single score on the above items.
9. Incapacitation due to abnormal movements.
   0 = none, normal
   1 = minimal
   2 = mild
   3 = moderate
   4 = severe
10. Patient's awareness of abnormal movements.
    0 = no awareness
    1 = aware, no distress
    2 = aware, mild distress
    3 = aware, moderate distress
    4 = aware, severe distress

Dental Status
11. Current problems with teeth and/or dentures.
    0 = no
    1 = yes
12. Does patient usually wear dentures?
    0 = no
    1 = yes

Reproduced from Guy W. ECDEU Assessment Manual for Psychopharmacology: Revised (DHEW publication number ADM 76-338). Rockville, MD, US Department of Health, Education and Welfare, Public Health Service, Alcohol, Drug Abuse and Mental Health Administration, NIMH Psychopharmacology Research Branch, Division of Extramural Research Programs, 1976: 534–7

Arizona Sexual Experiences Scale (ASEX)

Reference: **McGahuey CA, Gelenberg AJ, Laukes CA, Moreno FA, Delgado PL, McKnight KM, Manber R. The Arizona Sexual Experience Scale (ASEX): reliability and validity. Sex Marital Ther 2000; 26(1):25–40**

Rating Self-report

Administration time 5 minutes

Main purpose To measure sexual functioning

Population Adults

Commentary

The ASEX is a brief 5-item measure of sexual functioning, specifically, sexual drive, arousal, penile erection/vaginal lubrication, ability to reach orgasm and satisfaction with orgasm over the past week. The ASEX represents an easy-to-administer tool for assessing sexual dysfunction as a side-effect of pharmacological interventions in patients with depression or anxiety disorders. It is appropriate for use in either heterosexual or homosexual populations, regardless of availability of a sexual partner.

Scoring

Items are rated on a 6-point scale ranging from 1 (hyperfunction) through to 6 (hypofunction), providing a total score range of 5–30.

Versions

Gender-specific versions of the scale are available. A total score of >18 or a score of ≥5 (very difficult) on any single item is indicative of clinically significant sexual dysfunction.

Additional references

Atmaca M, Kuloglu M, Tezcan E, Buyukbayram A. Switching to tianeptine in patients with antidepressant-induced sexual dysfunction. Hum Psychopharmacol. 2003;18(4):277–80.

Westenberg HG, Stein DJ, Yang H, Li D, Barbato LM. A double-blind placebo-controlled study of controlled release fluvoxamine for the treatment of generalized social anxiety disorder. J Clin Psychopharmacol. 2004; 24(1):49–55.

Address for correspondence

Department of Psychiatry, College of Medicine
The University of Arizona
Arizona Health Sciences Center
1501 N. Campbell Ave, Tucson, AZ 85721, USA
Telephone: 1-520-626-7536
Email: meortiz@email.arizona.edu

Arizona Sexual Experiences Scale (ASEX) – Female

For each item, please indicate your **OVERALL** level during the **PAST WEEK**, including TODAY.

1. How strong is your sex drive?

1	2	3	4	5	6
extremely strong	very strong	somewhat strong	somewhat weak	very weak	no sex drive

2. How easily are you sexually aroused (turned on)?

1	2	3	4	5	6
extremely easily	very easily	somewhat easily	somewhat difficult	very difficult	nerer aroused

3. How easily does your vagina beome moist or wet during sex?

1	2	3	4	5	6
extremely easily	very easily	somewhat easily	somewhat difficult	very difficult	nerer aroused

4. How easily can you reach an orgasm?

1	2	3	4	5	6
extremely easily	very easily	somewhat easily	somewhat difficult	very difficult	nerer reach orgasm

5. Are your orgasms satisfying?

1	2	3	4	5	6
extremely satisfying	very satisfying	somewhat satisfying	somewhat unsatisfying	very unsatisfying	can't reach orgasm

COMMENTS:

Brief Pain Inventory (BPI)

Reference: Cleeland CS. Pain assessment in cancer. In: Osaba D (ed). Effect of Cancer on Quality of Life, Chapter 21. Boca Raton, FL, CRC Press, 1991

Rating Self-report

Administration time 5 minutes (short form), 10 minutes (long form)

Main purpose To assess the severity of pain and the impact of pain on daily functions

Population Adults

Commentary

The BPI (formerly the Wisconsin Brief Pain Questionnaire) is a comprehensive scale than assesses current pain, and pain at its worst, least and average over the previous week. Severity of pain, impact of pain on daily functioning, location of pain, pain medications, and amount of pain relief are assessed. Although initially developed to assess pain due to cancer, the BPI can be used to assess pain related to any medical condition, and provides a comprehensive assessment tool for evaluating pain in patients with depression or anxiety.

Scoring

Items are scored on a 0 (no pain) to 10 (pain as bad as you can imagine) scale. No scoring algorithm is used, but 'worst pain' or the mean of the 4 severity items can be used as a measure of pain severity and the mean of the 7 interference items can be used as a measure of pain interference.

Versions

The BPI has been translated into: Arabic, Cebuano, Chinese, Dutch, Filipino, French, German, Greek, Hindi, Italian, Japanese, Korean, Norwegian, Russian, Spanish, Swedish, Taiwanese and Vietnamese, and work is underway to translate the scale into Croatian, Czech, Hebrew, Portuguese, Slovene and Slovak. An Interactive Voice Response System (IVR) version is also available.

Additional references

Cleeland CS. Measurement of pain by subjective report. In: Chapman CR, Loeser JD (eds) Issues in Pain Measurement. New York: Raven Press 1989, pp 391–403. (Volume 12 of the series Advances in Pain Research and Therapy).

Cleeland CS, Gonin R, Hatfield AK, Edmonson JH, Blum RH, Stewart JA, Pandya KJ. Pain and its treatment in outpatients with metastatic cancer. N Engl J Med 1994; 330(9):592–6.

Tan G, Jensen MP, Thornby JI, Shanti BF. Validation of the brief pain inventory for chronic nonmalignant pain. J Pain 2004; 5(2):133–7.

Address for correspondence

Dr. Charles S. Cleeland
Department of Symptom Research
Box 221, 1515 Holcombe Blvd
Houston, TX 77030, USA
Telephone: 1-713-745-3470
Email: ccleeland@mdanderson.org

Brief Pain Inventory (Short Form)

Date:____/____/____ Time:_____

Name:_____

| Last | First | Middle Initial |

1. Throughout our lives, most of us have had pain from time to time (such as minor headaches, sprains, and toothaches). Have you had pain other than these everyday kinds of pain today?
   1. yes   2. no

2. On the diagram, shade in the areas where you feel pain. Put an X on the area that hurts the most.

3. Please rate your pain by circling the one number that best describes your pain at its WORST in the past 24 hours.

   0   1   2   3   4   5   6   7   8   9   10
   No   Pain as bad as
   pain   you can imagine

4. Please rate your pain by circling the one number that best describes your pain at its LEAST in the past 24 hours.

   0   1   2   3   4   5   6   7   8   9   10
   No   Pain as bad as
   pain   you can imagine

5. Please rate your pain by circling the one number that best describes your pain on the AVERAGE.

   0   1   2   3   4   5   6   7   8   9   10
   No   Pain as bad as
   pain   you can imagine

6. Please rate your pain by circling the one number that tells how much pain you have RIGHT NOW.

   0   1   2   3   4   5   6   7   8   9   10
   No   Pain as bad as
   pain   you can imagine

7. What treatments or medications are you receiving for your pain?

   _____

Brief Pain Inventory (Short Form)

8.   In the past 24 hours, how much RELIEF have pain treatments or medications provided? Please circle the one percentage that most shows how much relief you have received

0%	10%	20%	30%	40%	50%	60%	70%	80%	90%	100%
No relief										Complete relief

9.   Circle the one number that describes how, during the past 24 hours, PAIN HAS INTERFERED with your:

A. General Activity:

0	1	2	3	4	5	6	7	8	9	10
Does not interfere										Completely interferes

B. Mood

0	1	2	3	4	5	6	7	8	9	10
Does not interfere										Completely interferes

C. Walking ability

0	1	2	3	4	5	6	7	8	9	10
Does not interfere										Completely interferes

D. Normal work (includes both work outside the home and housework)

0	1	2	3	4	5	6	7	8	9	10
Does not interfere										Completely interferes

E. Relations with other people

0	1	2	3	4	5	6	7	8	9	10
Does not interfere										Completely interferes

F. Sleep

0	1	2	3	4	5	6	7	8	9	10
Does not interfere										Completely interferes

G. Enjoyment of life

0	1	2	3	4	5	6	7	8	9	10
Does not interfere										Completely interferes

Source: Pain Research Group, Department of Neurology, University of Wisconsin-Madison. Used with permission. May be duplicated and used in clinical practice.

Brief Psychiatric Rating Scale (BPRS)

Reference: **Overall JE, Gorham DR. The Brief Psychiatric Rating Scale. Psychol Rep 1962; 10:799–812**

Rating Clinician-rated

Administration time 10–30 minutes

Main purpose To assess psychiatric symptoms and severe psychopathology

Population Adults with psychiatric disorders

Commentary

The BPRS was designed to assess change in overall psychopathology in patients with a major psychiatric disorder, particularly psychosis. The instrument possesses 8 items that are rated on a 7-point scale by a trained interviewer and assesses a broad range of symptoms including thought disorder, withdrawal, anxiety-depression, hostility-suspicion, and activity. Ratings are categorized into those based on direct observation of the patient during the interview, or those based upon patient report for the previous 2 weeks. Completion times for the scale will vary widely according to the clinician's familiarity with the patient and the number of symptoms being rated. The BPRS remains one of the most widely used clinician-administered tools for evaluating baseline psychopathology and measuring change in psychotic and non-psychotic symptoms. It is less useful for patients with low levels of psychopathology, and training is required in its use (administration instructions are provided in Overall and Gorham, 1988).

Scoring

Symptom severity is rated on a 1 (absent) to 7 (extremely severe) scale; items are summed to produce a total pathology score.

Versions

A 21-item instrument for children called the BPRS-C is available, but is not related to the original BRPS. There is a modified version of the BPRS for nurses (BPRSNM), and the scale has been translated into: Czech, Danish, Dutch, French, German, Italian, Spanish and Turkish.

Additional references

Hedlund JL, Vieweg BW. The Brief Psychiatric Rating Scale (BPRS): A comprehensive review. Journal Operat Psychiatry 1980; 11:48–65.

Lukoff D, Liberman RP, Nuechterlein KH. Symptom monitoring in the rehabilitation of schizophrenic patients. Schizophr Bull 1986; 12(4):578–602.

Overall JE, Gorham DR. The Brief Psychiatric Rating Scale (BPRS): recent developments in ascertainment and scaling. Psychopharmacol Bull 1988; 24:97–9.

Silverstein ML, Mavrolefteros G, Close D. BPRS syndrome scales during the course of an episode of psychiatric illness. J Clin Psychol 1997; 53(5):455–8.

Address for correspondence

Dr. John E. Overall
Department of Psychiatry and Behavioural Sciences
University of Texas Medical School at Houston
PO Box 20708
Houston, TX 77225, USA
Telephone: 1-713-500-2500
Email: John.E.Overall@uth.tmc.edu

The Brief Psychiatric Rating Scale (BPRS)

This form consists of 18-symptom constructs, each to be rated on a 7-point scale of severity, ranging from 'not present' to 'extremely severe'. If a specific symptom is not rated, mark '0' = Not Assessed. Enter the score for the description which best describes the patient's condition.

0 = not assessed	3 = mild	6 = severe
1 = not present	4 = moderate	7 = extremely severe
2 = very mild	5 = moderately severe	

1. _____ **Somatic Concern:** Degree of concern over present bodily health. Rate the degree to which physical health is perceived as a problem by the patient, whether complaints have a realistic basis or not.

2. _____ **Anxiety:** Worry, fear, or overconcern for present or future. Rate solely on the basis of verbal report of patient's own subjective experiences. Do not infer anxiety from physical signs or from neurotic defense mechanisms.

3. _____ **Emotional Withdrawal:** Deficiency in relating to the interviewer and to the interviewer situation. Rate only the degree to which the patient gives the impression of failing to be in emotional contact with other people in the interview situation.

4. _____ **Conceptual Disorganization:** Degree to which the thought processes are confused, disconnected, or disorganized. Rate on the basis of integration of the verbal products of the patient; do not rate on the basis of patient's subjective impression of his own level of functioning.

5. _____ **Guilt Feelings:** Overconcern or remorse for past behavior. Rate on the basis of the patient's subjective experiences of guilt as evidenced by verbal report with appropriate affect; do not infer guilt feelings from depression, anxiety, or neurotic defenses.

6. _____ **Tension:** Physical and motor manifestations of tension, nervousness, and heightened activation level. Tension should be rated solely on the basis of physical signs and motor behavior and not on the basis of subjective experiences of tension reported by the patient.

7. _____ **Mannerisms and Posturing:** Unusual and unnatural motor behavior, the type of motor behavior which causes certain mental patients to stand out in a crowd of normal people. Rate only abnormality of movements; do not rate simple heightened motor activity here.

8. _____ **Grandiosity:** Exaggerated self-opinion, conviction of unusual ability or powers. Rate only on the basis of patient's statements about himself or self in relation to others, not on the basis of his demeanor in the interview situation.

9. _____ **Depressive Mood:** Despondency in mood, sadness. Rate only degree of despondency; do not rate on the basis of interferences concerning depression based upon general retardation and somatic complaints.

10. _____ **Hostility:** Animosity, contempt, belligerence, disdain for other people outside the interview situation. Rate solely on the basis of the verbal report of feelings and actions of the patient toward others; do not infer hostility from neurotic defenses, anxiety, nor somatic complaints. Rate attitude toward interviewer under 'uncooperativeness'.

11. _____ **Suspiciousness:** Belief, delusional or otherwise, that others have now or have had in the past, malicious or discriminatory intent toward the patient. On the basis of verbal report, rate only those suspicions which are currently held whether they concern past or present circumstances.

12. _____ **Hallucinatory Behavior:** Perceptions without normal external stimulus correspondence. Rate only those experiences which are reported to have occurred within the last week and which are described as distinctly different from the thought and imagery processes of normal people.

13. _____ **Motor Retardation:** Reduction in energy level evidenced by slow movements. Rate on the basis of observed behavior of the patient only; do not rate on the basis of patient's subjective impression of own energy level.

14. _____ **Uncooperativeness:** Evidence of resistance, unfriendliness, resentment, and lack of readiness to cooperate with interviewer. Rate only on the basis of the patient's attitude and responses to the interviewer, and interview situation; do not rate on the basis of reported resentment or uncooperativeness outside the interview situation.

15. _____ **Unusual Thought Content:** Unusual, odd, strange, or bizarre thought content. Rate here the degree of unusualness, not the degree of disorganization of thought processes.

16. _____ **Blunted Affect:** Reduced emotional tone, apparent lack of normal feeling or involvement.

17. _____ **Excitement:** Heightened emotional tone, agitation, increased reactivity.

18. _____ **Disorientation:** Confusion or lack of proper association for person, place, or time.

Reproduced with permission of authors and publisher from Overall JE, Gorham DR. Psychol Rep 1962; 10:799–812. © Southern Universities Press 1962.

Brief Symptom Inventory (BSI)

Reference: **Derogatis LR. Brief Symptom Inventory (BSI) Administration, Scoring, and Procedures Manual (3rd ed.). 1993. Minneapolis, MN, National Computer Systems**

Rating Self-report

Administration time 10 minutes

Main purpose To assess severity of psychological symptoms

Population Adults and adolescents

Commentary

The BSI (the self-report form of the Symptom Checklist-90-R, see page 166) is a 53-item measure designed to assess severity of psychological symptoms over the past week in psychiatric, medical or community samples. It yields 3 global domains (a global severity index, a positive symptom distress index and a positive symptom total) in addition to 9 symptom scales (somatization, obsessive-compulsive, interpersonal sensitivity, depression, anxiety, hostility, phobic anxiety, paranoid ideation and psychoticism). Norms are available for both psychiatric outpatient and inpatient populations. The BSI can be used to screen for psychological distress and has been used to assess response to treatment in a wide variety of clinical settings. An abbreviated 18-item version (the BSI 18) is also available.

Scoring

Items are scored on a 0–4 scale, with higher scores indicating greater symptom severity. Scoring can be performed manually or by computer. Scoring by hand involves the use of scoring templates and the conversion of raw scores, described in detail in the users' manual. The license holders provide a computerized scoring service, profile reports and narrative reports.

Versions

The scale has been translated into: Arabic, Canadian French, Chinese, Danish, Dutch, French, German, Hebrew, Italian, Japanese, Korean, Norwegian, Portuguese, Spanish, Swedish and Vietnamese.

Additional references

Derogatis LR, Melisaratos N. The Brief Symptom Inventory: an introductory report. Psychol Med 1983; 13(3):595–605.

Piersma HL, Boes JL. Agreement between patient self-report and clinician Rating concurrence between the BSI and the GAF among psychiatric inpatients. J Clin Psychol 1995; 51(2):153–7.

Allen JG, Coyne L, Huntoon J. Trauma pervasively elevates Brief Symptom Inventory profiles in inpatient women. Psychol Rep 1998; 83(2):499–513.

Address for correspondence

Pearson Assessments (formerly NCS Assessments)
Telephone: 1-800-627-7271, ext. 3225
or 1-952-681-3225
Fax: 1-800-632-9011 or 1-952-681-3299
Email: pearsonassessments@pearson.com
Website: www.pearsonassessments.com

Clinical Global Impression (CGI)

Reference: **Guy W, editor. ECDEU Assessment Manual for Psychopharmacology. 1976. Rockville, MD, U.S. Department of Health, Education, and Welfare**

Rating Clinician-rated

Administration time Varies with familiarity with patient

Main purpose To provide a global rating of illness severity, improvement and response to treatment

Population Adults

Commentary

Amongst the most widely used of extant brief assessment tools in psychiatry, the CGI is a 3-item observer-rated scale that measures illness severity (CGIS), global improvement or change (CGIC) and therapeutic response. The illness severity and improvement sections of the instrument are used more frequently than the therapeutic response section in both clinical and research settings. The Early Clinical Drug Evaluation Program (ECDEU) version of the CGI (reproduced here) is the most widely used format, and asks that the clinician rate the patient relative to their past experience with other patients with the same diagnosis, with or without collateral information. Several alternative versions of the CGI have been developed, however, such as the FDA Clinicians' Interview-Based Impression of Change (CIBIC), which uses only information collected during the interview, not collateral. The CGI has proved to be a robust measure of efficacy in many clinical drug trials, and is easy and quick to administer, provided that the clinician knows the patient well.

Scoring

The CGI is rated on a 7-point scale, with the severity of illness scale using a range of responses from 1 (normal) through to 7 (amongst the most severely ill patients). CGI-C scores range from 1 (very much improved) through to 7 (very much worse). Treatment response ratings should take account of both therapeutic efficacy and treatment-related adverse events and range from 0 (marked improvement and no side-effects) and 4 (unchanged or worse and side-effects outweigh the therapeutic effects). Each component of the CGI is rated separately; the instrument does not yield a global score.

Versions

CGI for bipolar disorder (CGI-BD), FDA Clinicians' Interview-Based Impression of Change (CIBIC), Clinicians' Interview-Based Impression of Change-Plus (CIBIC+), NYU CIBIC+, Parke-Davis Pharmaceuticals Clinical Interview-Based Impression (CIBI); the CGI has been translated into most languages.

Additional references

Leon AC, Shear MK, Klerman GL, Portera L, Rosenbaum JF, Goldenberg I. A comparison of symptom determinants of patient and clinician global ratings in patients with panic disorder and depression. J Clin Psychopharmacol 1993; 13(5):327–31.

Spearing MK, Post RM, Leverich GS, Brandt D, Nolen W. Modification of the Clinical Global Impressions (CGI) Scale for use in bipolar illness (BP): the CGI-BP. Psychiatry Res 1997; 73(3):159–71.

Zaider TI, Heimberg RG, Fresco DM, Schneier FR, Liebowitz MR. Evaluation of the clinical global impression scale among individuals with social anxiety disorder. Psychol Med 2003; 33(4):611–22.

Address for correspondence

Not applicable – the CGI is in the public domain.

Clinical Global Impression (CGI)

1. **Severity of illness**
   Considering your total clinical experience with this particular population, how mentally ill is the patient at this time?

   0 = Not assessed   4 = Moderately ill
   1 = Normal, not at all ill   5 = Markedly ill
   2 = Borderline mentally ill   6 = Severely ill
   3 = Mildly ill   7 = Among the most extremely ill patients

2. **Global improvement:** Rate total improvement whether or not, in your judgement, it is due entirely to drug treatment.
   Compared to his condition at admission to the project, how much has he changed?

   0 = Not assessed   4 = No change
   1 = Very much improved   5 = Minimally worse
   2 = Much improved   6 = Much worse
   3 = Minimally improved   7 = Very much worse

3. **Efficacy index:** Rate this item on the basis of **drug effect only**.
   Select the terms which best describe the degrees of therapeutic effect and side effects and record the number in the box where the two items intersect.
   EXAMPLE: Therapeutic effect is rated as 'Moderate' and side effects are judged 'Do not significantly interfere with patient's functioning'.

Therapeutic effect		Side effects			
		None	Do not significantly interfere with patient's functioning	Significantly interferes with patient's functioning	Outweighs therapeutic effect
Marked	Vast improvement. Complete or nearly complete remission of all symptoms	01	02	03	04
Moderate	Decided improvement. Partial remission of symptoms	05	06	07	08
Minimal	Slight improvement which doesn't alter status of care of patient	09	10	11	12
Unchanged or worse		13	14	15	16

Not assessed = 00

Reproduced from Guy W, editor. ECDEU Assessment Manual for Psychopharmacology. 1976. Rockville, MD, U.S. Department of Health, Education, and Welfare

Dartmouth COOP Functional Assessment Charts (COOP)

Reference: **Nelson E, Wasson J, Kirk J, Keller A, Clark D, Dietrich A, Stewart A, Zubkoff M. Assessment of function in routine clinical practice: description of the COOP Chart method and preliminary findings. J Chronic Dis 1987; 40 Suppl 1:55S–69S**

Rating Self-report

Administration time 5 minutes

Main purpose To assess general health status and functioning

Population Adults and adolescents

Commentary

The COOP consists of 9 highly visual charts designed to assess general health and functioning in primary care patients. The charts measure the domains of physical functioning, emotional functioning, overall health, change in health, pain, daily activities, social activities, social support and quality of life over the past 2–4 weeks. Advantages of the COOP include its brevity (each chart takes less than a minute to complete), practicality and ease of interpretation by patients, making it a useful screening tool for overall health status in busy clinical settings.

Scoring

Each chart is scored on a 5-point scale; as the charts assess separate dimensions of functioning, an overall score is not derived. A chart score of 4/5 indicates highly impaired functioning.

Versions

Adolescent charts are available, and the COOP has been translated into Chinese, Danish, Dutch, Finnish, French, German, Hebrew, Italian, Japanese, Norwegian, Portuguese, Slovak, Spanish, Swedish and Urdu.

Additional reference

Froom J, Schlager DS, Steneker S, Jaffe A. Detection of Major Depressive Disorder in Primary Care Patients. J Am Board Fam Pract 1993; 6(1):5–11.

Addresses for correspondence

Dartmouth COOP Project
Dartmouth Medical School
Butler Building, HB 7265
Hanover, NH 03755, USA
Telephone: 1-603-650-1220

FNX Corporation
1 Dorset Lane
Lebanon, NH 03766, USA
Telephone: 1-800-369-6669
Website: http://www.dartmouth.edu/~coopproj/ or www.howsyourhealth.org

Duke Health Profile (DUKE)

Reference: Parkerson GR Jr, Broadhead WE, Tse CK. The Duke Health Profile. A 17-item measure of health and dysfunction. Med Care 1990; 28(11):1056–72

Rating Self-report

Administration time 5 minutes

Main purpose To assess general health status and health-related quality of life

Population Adults

Commentary

The DUKE is a 17-item self-report measure of functional health status and health-related quality of life (HRQOL) designed for use in adult ambulatory primary care patients. The instrument contains 5 main sub-scales: physical health, mental health, social functioning, perceived health and disability. Several other sub-scales (i.e. general health, anxiety-depression, self-esteem) can also be derived from the scale's primary items. Parkerson et al. (1996) have reported that the DUKE's 7-item anxiety-depression sub-scale shows good ability to detect symptoms of anxiety and depression compared with the State Anxiety Inventory (see page 109) and the Center for Epidemiologic Studies Depression Scale (see page 14). The main strengths of the DUKE lie in its ability to provide a rapid self-report method for assessing general health status and HRQOL. However, it may also be suitable for use as a screening tool for anxiety and depression. In one study, the DUKE anxiety-depression sub-scale correctly identified 71% of cases of DSM-III-R diagnosed anxiety, and 82% of cases of major depression (Parkerson and Broadhead 1997).

Scoring

Items are scored on a 3-point scale (0–2) and transformed sub-scale scores range from 0–100 (where higher scores indicate good health, except for the dysfunction dimension, where high scores indicate poor health). Detailed scoring information is available at the website below or in the users' guide.

Versions

The Duke has been translated into: Afrikaans, Chinese (Taiwan), Dutch, Dutch (Belgium), English (United Kingdom), French, French (Canada), German, Italian, Korean, Norwegian, Polish, Portuguese, Spanish (Castillian), Spanish (Argentina, Chile, and Peru), Spanish (United States), and Swedish.

Additional references

Parkerson GR, Broadhead WE, Tse CK. Anxiety and depressive symptom identification using the Duke Health Profile. J Clin Epidemiol 1996; 49(1):85–93.

Parkerson GR Jr, Broadhead WE. Screening for anxiety and depression in primary care using the Duke Anxiety-Depression Scale (DUKE-AD). Fam Med 1997; 29(3):177–81.

Address for correspondence

Dr. George R. Parkerson Jr.
Department of Community and Family Medicine
Duke University Medical Centre
PO Box 2914
Durham, NC 27710, USA
Telephone: 1-919-681-3043
Fax: 1-919-668-5125
Email: parke001@mc.duke.edu
Website: http://healthmeasures.mc.duke.edu

Duke Health Profile

Date Today:_____   Name: _____   ID Number: _____

Date of Birth: _____   Female _____   Male _____

<u>INSTRUCTIONS:</u> Here are some questions about your health and feelings. Please read each question carefully and tick your best answer. You should answer the questions in your own way. There are no right or wrong answers.

		Yes, describes me exactly	Somewhat describes me	No, doesn't describe me at all
1.	I like who I am	_____	_____	_____
2.	I am not an easy person to get along with	_____	_____	_____
3.	I am basically a healthy person	_____	_____	_____
4.	I give up too easily	_____	_____	_____
5.	I have difficulty concentrating	_____	_____	_____
6.	I am happy with my family relationships	_____	_____	_____
7.	I am comfortable being around people	_____	_____	_____

<u>TODAY</u> would you have any physical trouble or difficulty:		None	Some	A lot
8.	Walking up a flight of stairs	_____	_____	_____
9.	Running the length of a football field	_____	_____	_____

DURING THE <u>PAST WEEK</u>: How much trouble have you had with:		None	Some	A lot
10.	Sleeping	_____	_____	_____
11.	Hurting or aching in any part of your body	_____	_____	_____
12.	Getting tired easily	_____	_____	_____
13.	Feeling depressed or sad	_____	_____	_____
14.	Nervousness	_____	_____	_____

DURING THE <u>PAST WEEK</u>: How often did you:		None	Some	A lot
15.	Socialize with other people (talk or visit with friends or relatives)	_____	_____	_____
16.	Take part in social, religious, or recreation activities (meetings, church, movies, sports, parties)	_____	_____	_____

DURING THE <u>PAST WEEK</u>: How often did you:		None	1–4 days	5–7 days
17.	Stay in your home, a nursing home, or hospital because of sickness, injury, or other health problem	_____	_____	_____

Reproduced from Parkerson GR Jr, Broadhead WE, Tse CK. Med Care 1990; 28(11):1056–72.
© 1989–2004 by the Department of Community and Family Medicine, Duke University Medical Center, Durham NC, USA.

Epworth Sleepiness Scale (ESS)

Reference: **Johns MW. A new method for measuring daytime sleepiness: the Epworth sleepiness scale. Sleep 1991; 14(6):540–5**

Rating Self-report

Administration time 5 minutes

Main purpose To assess levels of daytime sleepiness

Population Adults and older adults

Commentary

The ESS is an 8-item self-report questionnaire designed to assess levels of daytime sleepiness. The scale asks respondents to assess the likelihood of falling asleep in a number of common situations such as reading or watching television. ESS scores give a useful brief measure of average sleep propensity, and can be used as a screening tool to identify patients who require more detailed testing by techniques such as the multiple sleep latency test (MSLT).

Scoring

Items are rated on a 0 (would never doze) to 3 (high chance of dozing) scale, yielding a total score range of 0–24. Scores of >10 are suggestive of considerable daytime sleepiness; scores of >15 are associated with pathological sleepiness.

Versions

The scale has been translated into Chinese, Flemish, French, German, Italian, Portuguese, Spanish and Swedish. A computer-administered version is also available.

Additional references

Johns MW. Reliability and factor analysis of the Epworth Sleepiness Scale. Sleep 1992; 15(4):376–81.

Miletin MS, Hanly PJ. Measurement properties of the Epworth sleepiness scale. Sleep Med 2003; 4(3):195–9.

Address for correspondence

Dr. Murray W. Johns
Epworth Sleep Centre
Epworth Hospital
187 Hoddle Street
Richmond, Victoria 3121, Australia
Telephone: 61 3 9427 1849
Email: mwjohns@alphalink.com.au

Epworth Sleepiness Scale

Name: _____

Today's date: _____

Your age (years): _____

Your sex (Male = M, Female = F): _____

How likely are you to doze off or fall asleep in the following situations, in contrast to feeling just tired?

This refers to your usual way of life in recent times.

Even if you have not done some of these things recently try to work out how they would have affected you.

Use the following scale to choose the **most appropriate number** for each situation:

0 = would **never** doze
1 = **slight chance** of dozing
2 = **moderate chance** of dozing
3 = **high chance** of dozing

It is important that you answer each question as best you can.

Situation	Chance of dozing (0–3)
Sitting and reading	☐
Watching TV	☐
Sitting inactive in a public place (e.g a theatre or a meeting)	☐
As a passenger in a car for an hour without a break	☐
Lying down to rest in the afternoon when circumstances permit	☐
Sitting and talking to someone	☐
Sitting quietly after a lunch without alcohol	☐
In a car, while stopped for a few minutes in traffic	☐

Extrapyramidal Symptom Rating Scale (ESRS)

Reference: **Chouinard G, Ross-Chouinard A, Annable L, Jones BD. Extrapyramidal Symptom Rating Scale. Can J Neurol Sci 1980; 7:233**

Rating Clinician-rated and motor examination

Administration time 15 minutes

Main purpose To assess severity of extrapyramidal symptoms (Parkinsonism, akathisia, dystonia, dyskinesia)

Population Adults, adolescents and children

Commentary

The ESRS is a 12-item clinician-rated scale designed to assess the severity of extrapyramidal symptoms, including akathisia. Dyskinetic movements are rated according to both frequency and amplitude. The ESRS is widely used in clinical trials to assess extrapyramidal side-effects of antipsychotic medications, and its advantages are that it measures the four types of drug-induced movement disorders (parkinsonism, akathisia, dystonia and dyskinesia).

Scoring

Items are rated on a 7-point scale ranging from 0 (normal) through to 6 (extremely severe).

Versions

The ESRS has been translated into Croatian, Czech, English, French, German, Italian, Hungarian, Malayan, Mandarin, Portuguese, Spanish, Tugalog and Thai.

Additional references

Madhusoodanan S, Brenner R, Suresh P, Concepcion NM, Florita CD, Menon G, Kaur A, Nunez G, Reddy H. Efficacy and tolerability of olanzapine in elderly patients with psychotic disorders: a prospective study. Ann Clin Psychiatry 2000; 12(1):11–18.

Corya SA, Andersen SW, Detke HC, Kelly LS, Van Campen LE, Sanger TM, Williamson DJ, Dube S. Long-term antidepressant efficacy and safety of olanzapine/fluoxetine combination: a 76-week open-label study. J Clin Psychiatry 2003; 64(11):1349–56.

Tohen M, Goldberg JF, Gonzalez-Pinto Arrillaga AM, Azorin JM, Vieta E, Hardy-Bayle MC, Lawson WB, Emsley RA, Zhang F, Baker RW, Risser RC, Namjoshi MA, Evans AR, Breier A. A 12-week, double-blind comparison of olanzapine vs haloperidol in the treatment of acute mania. Arch Gen Psychiatry 2003; 60(12):1218–26.

Address for correspondence

Dr. Guy Chouinard
Allan Memorial Institute, McGill University and Centre de Recherche Fernand Séguin
Psychopharmacologie
Département de Psychiatrie
Université de Montréal
Hôpital Louis-Lafontaine
7401, rue Hochelaga
Montréal, Quebec H1N 3M5, Canada
Telephone: 1-514-251-4000 ext 3535
Email: guy.chouinard@umontreal.ca

EXTRAPYRAMIDAL SYMPTOM RATING SCALE (ESRS) (CHOUINARD) © 1979

The ESRS must be completed by the same rater throughout the whole study.

Date of assessment: (Day/Month/Year) |__|__| |__|__|__| |__|__| Raters Initials : |__|__|__|

In case of doubt please score the less severity.

I. PARKINSONISM, AKATHISIA, DYSTONIA AND DYSKINESIA : QUESTIONNAIRE

*In this questionnaire, take into account the verbal report of the patient on the following: 1) the duration of the symptom during the day; 2) the number of days where the symptom was present during **the last week**; and, 3) the evaluation of the intensity of the symptom by the patient.*

Enquire into the status of each symptom and rate accordingly.	Absent	Mild	Moderate	Severe	
1. Impression of slowness or weakness, difficulty in carrying out routine tasks	0	1	2	3	|__|
2. Difficulty walking or with balance.	0	1	2	3	|__|
3. Difficulty swallowing or talking	0	1	2	3	|__|
4. Stiffness, stiff posture	0	1	2	3	|__|
5. Cramps or pains in limbs, back or neck	0	1	2	3	|__|
6. Restless, nervous, unable to keep still	0	1	2	3	|__|
7. Tremors, shaking	0	1	2	3	|__|
8. Oculogyric crisis, abnormal sustained posture	0	1	2	3	|__|
9. Increased salivation	0	1	2	3	|__|
10. Abnormal involuntary movements (dyskinesia) of extremities or trunk	0	1	2	3	|__|
11. Abnormal involuntary movements (dyskinesia) of tongue, jaw, lips or face	0	1	2	3	|__|
12. Dizziness when standing up (especially in the morning)	0	1	2	3	|__|

II. PARKINSONISM and AKATHISIA : EXAMINATION
Items based on physical examinations for Parkinsonism.

1. Tremor

	Occasional	Frequent	Constant or almost so				
None: 0				Right upper limb			|__|
Borderline: 1				Left upper limb			|__|
Small amplitude :	2	3	4	Right lower limb			|__|
Moderate amplitude :	3	4	5	Left lower limb			|__|
Large amplitude :	4	5	6	Head	|__|	Jaw/Chin	|__|
				Tongue	|__|	Lips	|__|

2. Bradykinesia
0: normal
1: global impression of slowness in movements
2: definite slowness in movements
3: very mild difficulty in initiating movements |__|
4: mild to moderate difficulty in initiating movements
5: difficulty in starting or stopping any movement, or freezing on initiating voluntary act
6: rare voluntary movement, almost completely immobile

3. Gait & posture
0: normal
1: mild decrease of pendular arm movement
2: moderate decrease of pendular arm movement, normal steps
3: no pendular arm movement, head flexed, steps more or less normal |__|
4: stiff posture (neck, back) small step (shuffling gait)
5: more marked, festination or freezing on turning
6: triple flexion, barely able to walk

4. Postural stability
0: normal
1: hesitation when pushed but no retropulsion
2: retropulsion but recovers unaided
3: exaggerated retropulsion without falling |__|
4: absence of postural response, would fall if not caught by examiner
5: unstable while standing, even without pushing
6: unable to stand without assistance

5. Rigidity

0: normal muscle tone	Right upper limb	|__|
1: very mild, barely perceptible	Left upper limb	|__|
2: mild (some resistance to passive movements)	Right lower limb	|__|
3: moderate (definite resistance to passive movements)	Left lower limb	|__|
4: moderately severe (moderate resistance but still easy to move limb)		
5: severe (marked resistance with definite difficulty to move the limb)		
6: extremely severe (limb nearly frozen)		

Extrapyramidal Symptom Rating Scale (ESRS) (continued)

Items based on overall observation during examination for Parkinsonism.

6. Expressive automatic movements
(Facial mask/speech)
0: normal
1: very mild decrease in facial expressiveness
2: mild decrease in facial expressiveness
3: rare spontaneous smile, decrease blinking, voice slightly monotonous |__|
4: no spontaneous smile, staring gaze, low monotonous speech, mumbling
5: marked facial mask, unable to frown, slurred speech
6: extremely severe facial mask with unintelligible speech

7. Akathisia
0: absent
1: looks restless, nervous, impatient, uncomfortable
2: needs to move at least one extremity
3: often needs to move one extremity or to change position |__|
4: moves one extremity almost constantly if sitting, or stamps feet while standing
5: unable to sit down for more than a short period of time
6: moves or walks constantly

8. Sialorrhea
0: absent
1: very mild
2: mild
3: moderate: impairs speech |__|
4: moderately severe
5: severe
6: extremely severe: drooling

III. DYSTONIA : EXAMINATION AND OBSERVATION

1. Acute torsion dystonia
0: absent
1: very mild
2: mild
3: moderate
4: moderately severe
5: severe
6: extremely severe

Right upper limb: |__|
Left upper limb: |__|
Right lower limb: |__|
Left lower limb: |__|
Head |__| Jaw |__|
Tongue |__| Lips |__|
Eyes |__| Trunk |__|

2. Non acute or chronic or tardive dystonia
0: absent
1: very mild
2: mild
3: moderate
4: moderately severe
5: severe
6: extremely severe

Right upper limb: |__|
Left upper limb: |__|
Right lower limb: |__|
Left lower limb: |__|
Head |__| Jaw |__|
Tongue |__| Lips |__|
Eyes |__| Trunk |__|

IV. DYSKINETIC MOVEMENTS : EXAMINATION/OBSERVATION

	Occasional*	Frequent**	Constant or almost so	
1. Lingual movements (slow lateral or torsion movement of tongue)				
none : 0				
borderline : 1				
clearly present, within oral cavity :	2	3	4	
with occasional partial protrusion :	3	4	5	
with complete protrusion :	4	5	6	|__|
2. Jaw movements (lateral movement, chewing, biting, clenching)				
none : 0				
borderline : 1				
clearly present, small amplitude :	2	3	4	
moderate amplitude, but without mouth opening :	3	4	5	
large amplitude, with mouth opening :	4	5	6	|__|
3. Bucco-labial movements (puckering, pouting, smacking, etc.)				
none : 0				
borderline : 1				
clearly present, small amplitude :	2	3	4	
moderate amplitude, forward movement of lips :	3	4	5	
large amplitude; marked, noisy smacking of lips :	4	5	6	|__|
4. Truncal movements (involuntary rocking, twisting, pelvic gyrations)				
none : 0				
borderline : 1				
clearly present, small amplitude :	2	3	4	
moderate amplitude :	3	4	5	
greater amplitude :	4	5	6	|__|

		Occasional*	Frequent**	Constant or almost so

5. **Upper extremities (choreoathetoid movements only: arms, wrists, hands, fingers)**

none	: 0			
borderline	: I			
clearly present, small amplitude, movement of one limb	:	2	3	4
moderate amplitude, movement of one limb or movement of small amplitude involving two limbs	:	3	4	5
greater amplitude, movement involving two limbs	:	4	5	6 |___|

6. **Lower extremities (choreoathetoid movements only: legs, knees, ankles, toes)**

none	: 0			
borderline	: I			
clearly present, small amplitude, movement of one limb	:	2	3	4
moderate amplitude, movement of one limb or movement of small amplitude involving two limbs	:	3	4	5
greater amplitude, movement involving two limbs	:	4	5	6 |___|

7. **Other involuntary movements (swallowing, irregular respiration, frowning, blinking, grimacing, sighing, etc.)**

none	: 0			
borderline	: I			
clearly present, small amplitude	:	2	3	4
moderate amplitude	:	3	4	5
greater amplitude	:	4	5	6 |___|

SPECIFY :

* when activated or rarely spontaneous; ** frequently spontaneous and present when activated

V. CLINICAL GLOBAL IMPRESSION OF SEVERITY OF DYSKINESIA
Considering your clinical experience, how severe is the dyskinesia at this time?

0 : absent	3 : mild	6 : marked
I : borderline	4 : moderate	7 : severe
2 : very mild	5 : moderately severe	8 : extremely severe

|___|

VI. CLINICAL GLOBAL IMPRESSION OF SEVERITY OF PARKINSONISM
Considering your clinical experience, how severe is the parkinsonism at this time?

0 : absent	3 : mild	6 : marked
I : borderline	4 : moderate	7 : severe
2 : very mild	5 : moderately severe	8 : extremely severe

|___|

VII. CLINICAL GLOBAL IMPRESSION OF SEVERITY OF DYSTONIA
Considering your clinical experience, how severe is the dystonia at this time?

0 : absent	3 : mild	6 : marked
I : borderline	4 : moderate	7 : severe
2 : very mild	5 : moderately severe	8 : extremely severe

|___|

VIII. CLINICAL GLOBAL IMPRESSION OF SEVERITY OF AKATHISIA
Considering your clinical experience, how severe is the akathisia at this time?

0 : absent	3 : mild	6 : marked
I : borderline	4 : moderate	7 : severe
2 : very mild	5 : moderately severe	8 : extremely severe

|___|

IX. STAGE OF PARKINSONISM (Hoehn & Yahr)

0 : absent

I : unilateral involvement only, minimal or no functional impairment (stage I)

2 : bilateral or midline involvement, without impairment of balance (stage II)

3 : mildly to moderately disabling: first signs of impaired righting or postural reflex (unsteadiness as the patient turns or when he is pushed from standing equilibrium with the feet together and eyes closed), patient is physically capable of leading independent life (stage III)

4 : severely disabling : patient is still able to walk and stand unassisted but is markedly incapacitated (stage IV)

5 : confinement to bed or wheelchair (stage V)

|___|

Examiner: _____   Date:_____

Fatigue Severity Scale (FSS)

Reference: **Krupp LB, LaRocca NG, Muir-Nash J, Steinberg AD. The Fatigue Severity Scale. Arch Neurol 1989; 46(10):1121–3**

Rating Self-report

Administration time 5 minutes

Main purpose To assess severity of fatigue

Population Adults

Commentary

The FSS, originally developed to assess fatigue in multiple sclerosis and other related conditions, includes 9 items to measure disabling fatigue. The scale was specifically designed to differentiate fatigue from clinical depression.

Scoring

Items are scored on a 1–7 scale, with higher scores (range 7–63) indicating greater severity of fatigue.

Versions

The scale has been translated into: Dutch, German, Greek, Norwegian, Spanish and Turkish.

Additional references

Bakshi R, Shaikh ZA, Miletich RS, Czarnecki D, Dmochowski J, Henschel K, Janardhan V, Dubey N, Kinkel PR. Fatigue in multiple sclerosis and its relationship to depression and neurologic disability. Mult Scler 2000; 6(3):181–5.

DeBattista C, Doghramji K, Menza MA, Rosenthal MH, Fieve RR; Modafinil in Depression Study Group. Adjunct modafinil for the short-term treatment of fatigue and sleepiness in patients with major depressive disorder: a preliminary double-blind, placebo-controlled study. J Clin Psychiatry 2003;64(9):1057–64.

Address for correspondence

Dr. Lauren B. Krupp
Department of Neurology
State University of New York at Stony Brook
HSC T-12-20
Stony Brook, NY 11794-8121, USA
Telephone: 631-444-2599
Email: Lauren.Krupp@stonybrook.edu

Fatigue Severity Scale (FSS)

INSTRUCTIONS:
Below are a series of statements regarding your Fatigue. By Fatigue we mean a sense of tiredness, lack of energy or total body give-out. Please read each statement and choose a number from 1 to 7, where #1 indicates you completely <u>disagree</u> with the statement and #7 indicates you completely <u>agree</u>. Please answer these questions as they apply to the past **TWO WEEKS**.

	Completely Disagree						Completely Agree
1. My motivation is lower when I am fatigued	1	2	3	4	5	6	7
2. Exercise brings on my fatigue	1	2	3	4	5	6	7
3. I am easily fatigued	1	2	3	4	5	6	7
4. Fatigue interferes with my physical functioning	1	2	3	4	5	6	7
5. Fatigue causes frequent problems for me	1	2	3	4	5	6	7
6. My fatigue prevents sustained physical functioning	1	2	3	4	5	6	7
7. Fatigue interferes with carrying out certain duties and responsibilities	1	2	3	4	5	6	7
8. Fatigue is among my 3 most disabling symptoms	1	2	3	4	5	6	7
9. Fatigue interferes with my work, family, or social life	1	2	3	4	5	6	7

General Health Questionnaire (GHQ)

Reference: **Goldberg DP, Hillier VF. A scaled version of the General Health Questionnaire. Psychol Med 1979; 9(1):139–45**

Rating Self-report

Administration time Dependant on version

Main purpose To screen for psychiatric distress related to physical illness

Population Adults, adolescents and older adults

Commentary

The GHQ is a self-report screening instrument for psychiatric morbidity that is available in four main versions: a 60-item, 30-item (that does not contain questions relating to physical illness), 28-item (a scaled version that assesses somatic symptoms, anxiety and insomnia, social dysfunction and depression) and a 12-item version. Developed to assess the psychological components of ill health, the GHQ evaluates change in a patient's ability to perform daily functions over 'the past few weeks'. Where scaled sub-scores are required, the GHQ-28 should be used. The 60-item version provides a comprehensive assessment, but takes approximately 15 minutes to complete and may be too lengthy in highly impaired patients, where the GHQ-12 may be more appropriate. The instrument generally shows good ability to detect psychiatric disorders, although the developers note that it may have limited ability to detect certain symptoms of anxiety, particularly phobias. The GHQ remains a widely used and versatile tool to screen for psychological distress, although it should not be used in isolation for diagnostic purposes.

Scoring

Scoring method is dependent upon the version being used and is described in detail in the manual. The instrument developers suggest screening cut-off points of 11/12 for the GHQ-60, 4/5 for the GHQ-30, 4/5 for the GHQ-28 and 1/2/3 for the GHQ-12.

Versions

The GHQ has been translated into Chinese, Dutch, French, Italian, Japanese, Norwegian and Spanish, amongst other languages, contact nferNelson for further details.

Additional references

Clarke DM, Smith GC, Herrman HE. A comparative study of screening instruments for mental disorders in general hospital patients. Int J Psychiatry Med 1993; 23(4):323–37.

Goldberg DP, Gater R, Sartorius N, Ustun TB, Piccinelli M, Gureje O, Rutter C. The validity of two versions of the GHQ in the WHO study of mental illness in general health care. Psychol Med 1997; 27(1):191–7.

Schmitz N, Kruse J, Heckrath C, Alberti L, Tress W. Diagnosing mental disorders in primary care: the General Health Questionnaire (GHQ) and the Symptom Check List (SCL-90-R) as screening instruments. Soc Psychiatry Psychiatr Epidemiol 1999; 34(7):360–6.

Address for correspondence

nferNelson
The Chiswick Centre
414 Chiswick High Road
London W4 5TF, UK
Telephone: +44 (0) 20 8996 8444
Email: information@nfer-nelson.co.uk
Website: http://www.nfer-nelson.co.uk

Global Assessment of Functioning (GAF)

Reference: **Endicott J, Spitzer RL, Fleiss JL, Cohen J. The global assessment scale. A procedure for measuring overall severity of psychiatric disturbance. Arch Gen Psychiatry 1976; 33(6):766–71**

Rating Clinician-rated

Administration time Very brief after patient evaluation

Main purpose To measure global psychosocial functioning in patients with psychiatric disorders

Population Adults

Commentary

The GAF (previously the Global Assessment Scale or GAS), which constitutes Axis V of the DSM-IV classification system, assigns a numeric value (on a 1–100 scale) to psychosocial functioning. The rater is required to assess the functioning of the patient disregarding impairment arising from physical or environmental limitations using information from any clinical source (e.g. clinical assessment, collateral, medical records). The GAF has been used extensively to assess baseline levels of psychosocial functioning and to predict and evaluate outcome in a wide variety of patient populations. The main strengths of the GAF are its brevity, ease of administration, high reliability and sensitivity to change. Limitations include its subjective nature and the manner in which it confounds symptoms and functioning.

Scoring

The GAF is scored on a 1–100 scale, where 1 represents the hypothetically most impaired patient and 100 the hypothetically healthiest patient. The scale is divided into 10 equal 10-point intervals (e.g. 1–10, 11–20) that have clear anchor points; the use of intermediate scores is encouraged.

Versions

Children's GAS and GAF self-report; the GAF scale is available in every language into which the DSM-IV has been translated.

Additional references

Hall RC. Global assessment of functioning. A modified scale. Psychosomatics 1995; 36(3):267–75.

Jones SH, Thornicroft G, Coffey M, Dunn G. A brief mental health outcome scale-reliability and validity of the Global Assessment of Functioning (GAF). Br J Psychiatry 1995; 166(5):654–9.

Address for correspondence

The GAF is available as part of DSM-IV from:
The American Psychiatric Association
Diagnostic and Statistical Manual of Mental Disorders
1400 K. Street NW
Suite 1101
Washington, DC 20005, USA
Telephone: 1-703-907-7300
Email: apa@psych.org

DSM-IV-AXIS V: Global Assessment of Functioning Scale

Consider psychological, social, and occupational functioning on a hypothetical continuum of mental health illness. Do not include impairment in functioning due to physical (or environmental) limitations. Indicate appropriate code for the **LOWEST** level of functioning during the week of **POOREST** functioning in the past month. (Use intermediate levels when appropriate, e.g., 15, 68).

91 ⇔ 100   Superior functioning in a wide range of activities, life's problems never seem to get out of hand, is sought out by others because of his or her many positive qualities. No symptoms.

90 ⇔ 81   Absent or minimal symptoms (e.g., mild anxiety before an exam), good functioning in all areas, interested and involved in a wide range of activities, socially effective, generally satisfied members).

80 ⇔ 71   If symptoms are present, they are transient and expectable reactions to psychosocial stressors (e.g. difficulty concentrating after family argument); no more than slight impairment in social, occupational, school functioning (e.g., temporarily falling behind in school work).

70 ⇔ 61   Some mild symptoms (e.g., depressed mood and mild insomnia) **OR** some difficulty in social, occupational, or school functioning (e.g., occasional truancy, or theft within the household), but generally functioning pretty well, has some meaningful interpersonal relationships.

60 ⇔ 51   Moderate symptoms (e.g., flat affect and circumstantial speech, occasional panic attacks) **OR** moderate difficulty in social, occupational, or school functioning (e.g. few friends, conflicts with peers or co-workers).

50 ⇔ 41   Serious symptoms (e.g., suicidal ideation, severe obsessional rituals, frequent shoplifting) **OR** any serious impairment in social, occupational, or school functioning (e.g., no friends, unable to keep a job).

40 ⇔ 31   Some impairment in reality testing or communication (e.g., speech is at times illogical, obscure, or irrelevant) **OR** major impairment in several areas, such as work or school, family relations, judgment, thinking, or mood (e.g., depressed man avoids friends, neglects family, and is unable to work; child frequently beats up younger children, is defiant at home, and is failing at school).

30 ⇔ 21   Behavior is considerably influenced by delusions or hallucinations **OR** serious impairment in communication or judgment (e.g., sometimes incoherent, acts grossly inappropriately, suicidal preoccupation) **OR** inability to function in almost all areas (e.g., stays in bed all day, no job, home, or friends).

20 ⇔ 11   Some danger of hurting self or others (e.g., suicide attempts without clear expectation of death; violent; manic excitement) **OR** occasionally fails to maintain minimal personal hygiene (e.g., smears feces) **OR** gross impairment in communication (e.g., largely incoherent or mute).

10 ⇔ 1   Persistent danger of severely hurting self or others (e.g., recurrent violence) **OR** persistent inability to maintain minimal personal hygiene **OR** serious suicidal act with clear expectation of death.

0   Inadequate information

Medical Outcomes Study Short-Form 36 (SF-36)

Reference: **Ware JE, Snow KK, Kosinski M, Gandek B. SF-36 Health Survey: Manual and Interpretation Guide. 1993. Boston, MA, The Health Institute**

Rating Self-report

Administration time 10 minutes

Main purpose To assess perceived health status

Population Adults and adolescents

Commentary

The SF-36 is a widely used self-report measure of generic (as opposed to disease-specific) health status. The instrument was designed to assess both physical and emotional well-being in a range of community and patient populations, clinical diagnoses and settings. The instrument evaluates how the individual has functioned over the previous 4 weeks in 8 primary domains: physical functioning, physical role limitation, bodily pain, social functioning, mental health, emotional role limitation, vitality (energy versus fatigue) and general health perceptions. A number of other versions of the scale are also available including the original SF-20, a 12-item scale and the newly developed SF-8, although the 36-item version remains the most commonly used version in both research and clinical settings. The SF-36 has been used extensively to assess health status and health-related quality of life in patients with mood and anxiety disorders. It represents the gold standard of generic health status measures, although instruments such as the Quality of Life Enjoyment and Satisfaction Questionnaire or Q-LES-Q (see page 150) may provide more clinically useful information in psychiatric populations.

Scoring

Items on the SF-36 are scored in a yes/no fashion, and on 3, 5 and 6-point scales. The 8 sub-scales have score ranges of 0–100, where higher scores indicate better health status. The instrument also yields physical and mental health summary scores.

Versions

The scale developers recommend using the SF-36 version 2.0 developed in 1996. An acute version that assesses functioning over the previous week (as opposed to 4 weeks) is also available. The International Quality of Life Assessment (IQOLA) Project is translating the SF-36 into a multitude of languages (see the Medical Outcomes Trust website for up-to-date information).

Additional references

Ware JE, Sherbourne CD. The Mos 36-Item Short-Form Health Survey (SF-36). 1. Conceptual-Framework and Item Selection. Med Care 1992; 30(6):473–83.

Wells KB, Burnam MA, Rogers W, Hays R, Camp P. The course of depression in adult outpatients: results from the Medical Outcomes Study. Arch Gen Psychiatry 1992; 49:788–94.

Hays RD, Wells KB, Sherbourne CD, Rogers W, Spritzer K. Functioning and well-being outcomes of patients with depression compared with chronic general medical illnesses. Arch Gen Psychiatry 1995; 52(1):11–19.

Address for correspondence

Permission to use the SF-36 must be obtained from the Medical Outcomes Trust:
Medical Outcomes Trust
235 Wyman St., Suite 130
Waltham, MA 02451, USA
Telephone: 1-781-890-4884
Email: info@outcomes-trust.org
Website: www.outcomes-trust.org

Pittsburgh Sleep Quality Index (PSQI)

Reference: **Buysse DJ, Reynolds CF 3rd, Monk TH, Berman SR, Kupfer DJ. The Pittsburgh Sleep Quality Index: a new instrument for psychiatric practice and research. Psychiatry Res 1989; 28(2):193–213**

Rating Self-report

Administration time 5–10 minutes

Main purpose To assess levels of daytime sleepiness and sleep disturbance

Population Adults, adolescents and older adults

Commentary

The PSQI is a 19-item self report instrument developed to assess sleep quality over the previous month (the scale also contains 5 items that can be rated in combination with the patient's partner, but these are not used when scoring the scale). The scale assesses several domains of sleep quality, including: subjective sleep quality, sleep latency, sleep duration, habitual sleep efficiency, sleep disturbances, use of sleep medications and daytime dysfunction. Patients with depression and anxiety disorders (e.g. panic disorder, social phobia as well as sleep disorders) have been shown to score higher on the scale than healthy control subjects. The PSQI represents a brief, clinically useful assessment of a variety of sleep disturbances that might affect sleep quality and can be used as a screening tool to identify good and poor sleepers. Several studies have documented the treatment responsiveness of PSQI.

Scoring

The majority of the scale's items are scored on a 0 (no difficulty) to 3 (severe difficulty) scale with 4 text questions that ask about usual bed and wake times, sleep latency and duration. The scale yields 7 component scores, and a global score with a range of 0–21; a global score of ≥5 suggests significant sleep disturbance.

Versions

The PSQI has been, or is in the process of being, translated into: Chinese, Dutch, Estonian, French for Canada, German, Hungarian, Japanese, Korean, Latvian, Lithuanian, Norwegian, Polish, Romanian, Russian, Spanish, Swedish, Taiwanese and Turkish.

Additional references

Stein MB, Chartier M, Walker JR. Sleep in nondepressed patients with panic disorder: I. Systematic assessment of subjective sleep quality and sleep disturbance. Sleep 1993; 16(8):724–6.

Stein MB, Kroft CD, Walker JR. Sleep impairment in patients with social phobia. Psychiatry Res 1993; 49(3):251–6.

Agargun MY, Kara H, Solmaz M. Subjective sleep quality and suicidality in patients with major depression. J Psychiatr Res 1997; 31(3):377–81.

Buysse DJ, Tu XM, Cherry CR, Begley AE, Kowalski J, Kupfer DJ, Frank E. Pretreatment REM sleep and subjective sleep quality distinguish depressed psychotherapy remitters and nonremitters. Biol Psychiatry 1999; 15;45(2):205–13.

Address for correspondence

Dr. Daniel J. Buysse
Western Psychiatric Institute & Clinic
University of Pittsburgh
3811 O'Hara Street
Pittsburgh, PA 15213, USA
Telephone: 1-412-246-6413
Email: buyssedj@upmc.edu

Pittsburgh Sleep Quality Index

INSTRUCTIONS:

The following questions relate to your usual sleep habits during the past month <u>only</u>. Your answers should indicate the most accurate reply for the <u>majority</u> of days and nights in the past month.

Please answer all questions.

1. During the past month, what time have you usually gone to bed at night?

    BED TIME _____

2. During the past month, how long (in minutes) has it usually taken you to fall asleep each night?

    NUMBER OF MINUTES _____

3. During the past month, what time have you usually gotten up in the morning?

    GETTING UP TIME _____

4. During the past month, how many hours of actual sleep did you get at night? (This may be different than the number of hours you spent in bed.)

    HOURS OF SLEEP PER NIGHT _____

For each of the remaining questions, check the one best response. Please answer <u>all</u> questions.

5. During the past month, how often have you had trouble sleeping because you ...

    a) Cannot get to sleep within 30 minutes

Not during the past month___	Less than once a week___	Once or twice a week___	Three or more times a week___

    b) Wake up in the middle of the night or early morning

Not during the past month___	Less than once a week___	Once or twice a week___	Three or more times a week___

    c) Have to get up to use the bathroom

Not during the past month___	Less than once a week___	Once or twice a week___	Three or more times a week___

    d) Cannot breathe comfortably

Not during the past month___	Less than once a week___	Once or twice a week___	Three or more times a week___

    e) Cough or snore loudly

Not during the past month___	Less than once a week___	Once or twice a week___	Three or more times a week___

    f) Feel too cold

Not during the past month___	Less than once a week___	Once or twice a week___	Three or more times a week___

    g) Feel too hot

Not during the past month___	Less than once a week___	Once or twice a week___	Three or more times a week___

    h) Had bad dreams

Not during the past month___	Less than once a week___	Once or twice a week___	Three or more times a week___

    i) Have pain

Not during the past month___	Less than once a week___	Once or twice a week___	Three or more times a week___

    j) Other reason(s), please describe _____

    _____

    How often during the past month have you had trouble sleeping because of this?

Not during the past month _____	Less than once a week _____	Once or twice a week _____	Three or more times a week _____

6. During the past month, how would you rate your sleep quality overall?

    Very good _____

    Fairly good _____

    Fairly bad _____

    Very bad _____

7. During the past month, how often have you taken medicine to help you sleep (prescribed or 'over the counter')?

Not during the past month _____	Less than once a week _____	Once or twice a week _____	Three or more times a week _____

8. During the past month, how often have you had trouble staying awake while driving, eating meals, or engaging in social activity?

Not during the past month _____	Less than once a week _____	Once or twice a week _____	Three or more times a week _____

9. During the past month, how much of a problem has it been for you to keep up enough enthusiasm to get things done?

      No problem at all   _____

      Only a very slight problem   _____

      Somewhat of a problem   _____

      A very big problem   _____

10. Do you have a bed partner or room mate?

      No bed partner or room mate   _____

      Partner/room mate in other room   _____

      Partner in same room, but not same bed _____

      Partner in same bed   _____

If you have a room mate or bed partner, ask him/her how often in the past month you have had ...

a) Loud snoring

| Not during the past month ___ | Less than once a week ___ | Once or twice a week ___ | Three or more times a week ___ |

b) Long pauses between breaths while asleep

| Not during the past month ___ | Less than once a week ___ | Once or twice a week ___ | Three or more times a week ___ |

c) Legs twitching or jerking while you sleep

| Not during the past month ___ | Less than once a week ___ | Once or twice a week ___ | Three or more times a week ___ |

d) Episodes of disorientation or confusion during sleep

| Not during the past month ___ | Less than once a week ___ | Once or twice a week ___ | Three or more times a week ___ |

e) Other restlessness while you sleep; please describe _____

| Not during the past month ___ | Less than once a week ___ | Once or twice a week ___ | Three or more times a week ___ |

Positive and Negative Syndrome Scale (PANSS)

Reference: **Kay SR, Opler LA, Fiszbein A. Positive and Negative Syndrome Scale Manual. 1994. North Tonawanda, NY, Multi-Health Systems Inc.**

Rating Clinician-administered

Administration time 30–40 minutes

Main purpose To assess severity of positive and negative symptoms in psychotic disorders

Population Adults and adolescents

Commentary

The PANSS is a 30-item clinician-administered scale designed to measure severity of symptoms in patients with schizophrenia, schizoaffective disorder, and other psychotic disorders over the past week. The instrument contains 3 sub-scales: a 7-item positive scale (assessing symptoms such as hallucinations and delusions), a 7-item negative scale (assessing symptoms such as blunted affect and social withdrawal) and a 16-item general psychopathology scale. Advantages of the PANSS include its broad evaluation (it assesses symptoms such as anxiety, guilt and depression in addition to positive and negative symptoms), provision of detailed anchor points to improve inter-rater reliability, and strong psychometric properties, particularly in terms of monitoring treatment response. Disadvantages of the instrument include its lengthy administration time, which may make it unsuitable for use in patients with cognitive dysfunction.

Scoring

Items are scored on a 7-point scale. Total scores for the positive and negative sub-scale range between 7 and 49, whereas the general psychopathology sub-scales has a score range of 16–112. A composite scale score can also be derived by subtracting the negative score from the positive score to indicate whether the patient's symptoms are predominantly positive or negative (range -42, only negative symptoms, to +42, only positive symptoms).

Versions

A child version of the scale, the Kiddie-PANSS, has been developed for children aged between 6–16 years, as well as a semi-structured interview version (the Structured Clinical Interview for the Positive and Negative Syndrome Scale or SCI-PANSS). The instrument has been translated into a wide variety of languages, including: Chinese, Danish, Dutch, Finnish, French, German, Italian, Polish, Spanish, Swedish and Thai.

Additional references

Kay SR, Fiszbein A, Opler LA. The positive and negative syndrome scale (PANSS) for schizophrenia. Schizophr Bull 1987; 13(2):261–76.

Bell M, Milstein R, Beam-Goulet J, Lysaker P, Cicchetti D. The Positive and Negative Syndrome Scale and the Brief Psychiatric Rating Scale. Reliability, comparability, and predictive validity. J Nerv Ment Dis 1992; 180(11):723–8.

Opler LA, Kay SR, Lindenmayer JP, Fiszbein A. Structured Clinical Interview for the Positive and Negative Syndrome Scale (SCI-PANSS). 1992. Toronto, Canada, Multi-Health Systems Inc.

Address for correspondence

Multi-Health Systems Inc.
P.O. Box 950
North Tonawanda, NY 14120-0950, USA
Telephone: 1-800-456-3003 in the US
or 1-416-492-2627 international
Email: customerservice@mhs.com
Website: www.mhs.com

Primary Care Evaluation of Mental Disorders Patient Health Questionnaire (PHQ)

Reference: Spitzer RL, Kroenke K, Williams JB. Validation and utility of a self-report version of PRIME-MD: the PHQ primary care study. Primary Care Evaluation of Mental Disorders. Patient Health Questionnaire. JAMA 1999; 282(18):1737–44

Rating Self-report

Administration time Depends on version

Main purpose To assess mental disorders, functional impairment, and recent psychosocial stressors

Population Adults

Commentary

The PHQ, a self-report version of the PRIME-MD interview, is a 4-page questionnaire. The first 3 pages assess common mental disorders (somatoform, mood, anxiety, eating, alcohol) and functional impairment. Many clinicians use only these first 3 pages, or components such as the popular 9-item depression module (the PHQ-9, see page 44). The fourth page includes questions about recent stressors and for women, questions regarding menstruation, pregnancy and childbirth. A 2-page version of the PHQ (the Brief PHQ) is available that assesses depression, anxiety, psychosocial stressors and some women's reproductive health issues, as is a PHQ-15 that assesses severity of somatic symptoms.

Scoring

Scoring methods are described in the Quick Guide to PRIME-MD Patient Health Questionnaire (PHQ) document (available from authors).

Versions

An adolescent version is available (PHQ-A) and the PHQ has been translated into: Chinese, French, German, Greek, Italian, Spanish and Vietnamese. A telephone scoring version is available from the authors, as is a slightly modified version that has additional questions about drug and alcohol use.

Additional references

Spitzer RL, Williams JBW, Kroenke K, Hornyak R, McMurray J. Validity and utility of the Patient Health Questionnaire in assessment of 3000 obstetrics-gynecologic patients. Am J Obstet Gynecol 2000; 183(3):759–69.

Johnson JG, Harris ES, Spitzer RL, Williams JB. The patient health questionnaire for adolescents: validation of an instrument for the assessment of mental disorders among adolescent primary care patients. J Adolesc Health 2002; 30(3):196–204.

Lowe B, Grafe K, Zipfel S, Spitzer RL, Herrmann-Lingen C, Witte S, Herzog W. Detecting panic disorder in medical and psychosomatic outpatients. Comparative validation of the Hospital Anxiety and Depression Scale, the Patient Health Questionnaire, a screening question, and physicians' diagnosis. Psychosom Res 2003; 55(6):515–19.

Address for correspondence

Dr. Robert L. Spitzer
Columbia University
1051 Riverside Drive, Unit 60
NYS Psychiatric Institute
New York, NY 10032, USA
Telephone: 1-212-543-5524
Email: RLS8@Columbia.edu

The PHQ is a trademark of Pfizer Inc.

Patient Health Questionnaire (PHQ)

This questionnaire is an important part of providing you with the best health care possible. Your answers will help in understanding problems that you may have. Please answer every question to the best of your ability unless you are requested to skip over a question.

Name _____ Age_____ Sex: ☐ Female ☐ Male Today's Date _____

1. During the <u>last 4 weeks</u>, how much have you been bothered by any of the following problems?

	Not bothered	Bothered a little	Bothered a lot
a. Stomach pain	☐	☐	☐
b. Back pain	☐	☐	☐
c. Pain in your arms, legs, or joints (knees, hips, etc.)	☐	☐	☐
d. Menstrual cramps or other problems with your periods	☐	☐	☐
e. Pain or problems during sexual intercourse	☐	☐	☐
f. Headaches	☐	☐	☐
g. Chest pain	☐	☐	☐
h. Dizziness	☐	☐	☐
i. Fainting spells	☐	☐	☐
j. Feeling your heart pound or race	☐	☐	☐
k. Shortness of breath	☐	☐	☐
l. Constipation, loose bowels, or diarrhea	☐	☐	☐
m. Nausea, gas, or indigestion	☐	☐	☐

2. Over the <u>last 2 weeks</u>, how often have you been bothered by any of the following problems?

	Not at all	Several days	More than half the days	Nearly every day
a. Little interest or pleasure in doing things	☐	☐	☐	☐
b. Feeling down, depressed, or hopeless	☐	☐	☐	☐
c. Trouble falling or staying asleep, or sleeping too much	☐	☐	☐	☐
d. Feeling tired or having little energy	☐	☐	☐	☐
e. Poor appetite or overeating	☐	☐	☐	☐
f. Feeling bad about yourself, or that you are a failure, or have let yourself or your family down	☐	☐	☐	☐
g. Trouble concentrating on things, such as reading the newspaper or watching television	☐	☐	☐	☐
h. Moving or speaking so slowly that other people could have noticed? Or the opposite – being so fidgety or restless that you have been moving around a lot more than usual	☐	☐	☐	☐
i. Thoughts that you would be better off dead, or of hurting yourself in some way	☐	☐	☐	☐

3. Questions about anxiety.

	No	Yes
a. In the <u>last 4 weeks</u>, have you had an anxiety attack – suddenly feeling fear or panic?	☐	☐

If you checked 'NO', go to question 5.

	No	Yes
b. Has this ever happened before?	☐	☐
c. Do some of these attacks come <u>suddenly out of the blue</u> that is, in situations where you don't expect to be nervous or uncomfortable?	☐	☐
d. Do these attacks bother you a lot or are you worried about having another attack?	☐	☐

4. Think about your last bad anxiety attack.

	No	Yes
a. Were you short of breath?	☐	☐
b. Did your heart race, pound, or skip?	☐	☐
c. Did you have chest pain or pressure?	☐	☐
d. Did you sweat?	☐	☐
e. Did you feel as if you were choking?	☐	☐
f. Did you have hot flashes or chills?	☐	☐
g. Did you have nausea or an upset stomach, or the feeling that you were going to have diarrhea?	☐	☐
h. Did you feel dizzy, unsteady, or faint?	☐	☐
i. Did you have tingling or numbness in parts of your body?	☐	☐
j. Did you tremble or shake?	☐	☐
k. Were you afraid you were dying?	☐	☐

Patient Health Questionnaire (PHQ)

5. Over the last 4 weeks, how often have you been bothered by any of the following problems?

	Not at all	Several days	More than half the days
a. Feeling nervous, anxious, on edge, or worrying a lot about different things	☐	☐	☐

If you checked 'Not at all', go to question 6

	Not at all	Several days	More than half the days
b. Feeling restless so that it is hard to sit still	☐	☐	☐
c. Getting tired very easily	☐	☐	☐
d. Muscle tension, aches, or soreness	☐	☐	☐
e. Trouble falling asleep or staying asleep	☐	☐	☐
f. Trouble concentrating on things, such as reading a book or watching TV	☐	☐	☐
g. Becoming easily annoyed or irritable	☐	☐	☐

6. Questions about eating.

	No	Yes
a. Do you often feel that you can't control <u>what</u> or <u>how much</u> you eat?	☐	☐
b. Do you often eat, <u>within any 2-hour period</u>, what most people would regard as an unusually <u>large</u> amount of food?	☐	☐

If you checked 'NO' to either a or b, go to question 9

	No	Yes
c. Has this been as often, on average, as twice a week for the last 3 months?	☐	☐

7. In the last 3 months have you <u>often</u> done any of the following in order to avoid gaining weight?

	No	Yes
a. Made yourself vomit?	☐	☐
b. Took more than twice the recommended dose of laxatives?	☐	☐
c. Fasted (not eaten anything at all for at least 24 hours)?	☐	☐
d. Exercised for more than an hour, specifically to avoid gaining weight after binge eating?	☐	☐

8. If you checked 'YES' to any of these ways of avoiding gaining weight, were any as often, on average, as twice a week?

	No	Yes
	☐	☐

9. Do you ever drink alcohol (including beer or wine)?

	No	Yes
	☐	☐

If you checked 'NO' go to question 11

10. Have any of the following happened to you <u>more than once in the last 6 months</u>?

	No	Yes
a. You drank alcohol even though a doctor suggested that you stop drinking because of a problem with your health	☐	☐
b. You drank alcohol, were high from alcohol, or hung over while you were working, going to school, or taking care of children or other responsibilities	☐	☐
c. You missed or were late for work, school, or other activities because you were drinking or hung over	☐	☐
d. You had a problem getting along with other people while you were drinking	☐	☐
e. You drove a car after having several drinks or after drinking too much	☐	☐

11. If you checked off <u>any</u> problems on this questionnaire, how <u>difficult</u> have these problems made it for you to do your work, take care of things at home, or get along with other people?

☐ **Not difficult at all**   ☐ **Somewhat difficult**   ☐ **Very difficult**   ☐ **Extremely difficult**

12. In the <u>last 4 weeks</u>, how much have you been bothered by any of the following problems?

	Not bothered	Bothered a little	Bothered a lot
a. Worrying about your health	☐	☐	☐
b. Your weight or how you look	☐	☐	☐
c. Little or no sexual desire or pleasure during sex	☐	☐	☐
d. Difficulties with husband/wife, partner/lover or boyfriend/girlfriend	☐	☐	☐
e. The stress of taking care of children, parents, or other family members	☐	☐	☐
f. Stress at work outside of the home or at school	☐	☐	☐
g. Financial problems or worries	☐	☐	☐
h. Having no one to turn to when you have a problem	☐	☐	☐
i. Something bad that happened <u>recently</u>	☐	☐	☐
j. Thinking or dreaming about something terrible that happened to you <u>in the past</u> – like your house being destroyed, a severe accident, being hit or assaulted, or being forced to commit a sexual act	☐	☐	☐

13. In the <u>last year</u>, have you been hit, slapped, kicked or otherwise physically hurt by someone, or has anyone forced you to have an unwanted sexual act?

No	Yes
☐	☐

14. What is the most stressful thing in your life right now? _____

_____

15. Are you taking any medicine for anxiety, depression or stress?

No	Yes
☐	☐

16. **FOR WOMEN ONLY: Questions about menstruation, pregnancy and childbirth.**

   a. Which best describes your menstrual periods?

☐ Periods are unchanged	☐ No periods because pregnant or recently gave birth	☐ Periods have become irregular or changed in frequency, duration or amount	☐ No periods for at least a year	☐ Having periods because taking hormone replacement (estrogen) therapy or oral contraceptive

   b. During the week before your period starts, do you have a <u>serious</u> problem with your mood – like depression, anxiety, irritability, anger or mood swings?

	No (or does not apply)	Yes
b.	☐	☐
c. If YES: Do these problems go away by the end of your period?	☐	☐
d. Have you given birth within the last 6 months?	☐	☐
e. Have you had a miscarriage within the last 6 months?	☐	☐
f. Are you having difficulty getting pregnant?	☐	☐

Developed by Drs. Robert L. Spitzer, Janet B.W. Williams, Kurt Kroenke and colleagues, with an educational grant from Pfizer Inc. For research information, contact Dr. Spitzer at rls8@columbia.edu. The names PRIME-MD® and PRIME-MD TODAY® are trademarks of Pfizer Inc.
© 1999, Pfizer Inc.

Profile of Mood States (POMS)

Reference: **McNair DM, Lorr M, Droppleman LF. EdITS Manual for the Profile of Mood States. 1992. San Diego, CA, EdITS**

Rating Self-report

Administration time <5 minutes

Main purpose To assess mood state and changes in mood

Population Adults

Commentary

The POMS is a 65-item self-report questionnaire designed to assess mood state over the previous week or for shorter periods such as 'right now'. Each item consists of an adjective, some of which reflect positive mood states (for example, lively, cheerful, clear-headed), whereas others reflect negative mood states (for example, sad, unhappy, hopeless). The scale assesses 6 main domains: Tension-Anxiety, Depression-Dejection, Anger-Hostility, Vigour-Activity, Fatigue-Inertia and Confusion-Bewilderment. The POMS is quick and easy to administer and has a long history of use as an outcome instrument, particularly in studies requiring a measure that is sensitive to transient, fluctuating affective mood states.

Scoring

Items are scored on a 0 (not at all) to 4 (extremely) basis; the total mood score (range 0–260) is obtained by summing the scores of the 5 negative mood scales, but discounting the Vigour scale. The 6 sub-scales are derived by summing the scores for the relevant adjectives.

Versions

A 30-item short form is available, as well as a bipolar supplement. The instrument has been translated into: Chinese, Czech, Danish, Dutch, Finnish, French, German, Greek, Italian, Japanese, Norwegian, Polish, Russian, Spanish and Swedish.

Additional references

Szuba MP, Baxter LR Jr, Fairbanks LA, Guze BH, Schwartz JM. Effects of partial sleep deprivation on the diurnal variation of mood and motor activity in major depression. Biol Psychiatry 1991; 30(8):817–29.

Nyenhuis DL, Yamamoto C, Luchetta T, Terrien A, Parmentier A. Adult and geriatric normative data and validation of the profile of mood states. J Clin Psychol 1999; 55(1):79–86.

Address for correspondence

Multi-Health Systems Inc.
P.O. Box 950
North Tonawanda, NY 14120-0950, USA
Telephone: 1-800-456-3003 in the US
or 1-416-492-2627 international
Email: customerservice@mhs.com
Website: www.mhs.com

Quality of Life Enjoyment and Satisfaction Questionnaire (Q-LES-Q)

Reference: **Endicott J, Nee J, Harrison W, Blumenthal R. Quality of Life Enjoyment and Satisfaction Questionnaire: a new measure. Psychopharmacol Bull 1993; 29(2):321–6**

Rating Self-report

Administration time 10 minutes

Main purpose To assess generic quality of life

Population Adults

Commentary

The Q-LES-Q is a 93-item self-report measure of generic quality of life that was developed in a population of outpatients with depression. The scale possesses 8 sub-scales (physical health, work, school, household duties, subjective feelings, leisure activities, social relationships and general activities), although completion of the work, school and household duties sections is optional. The Q-LES-Q is fast becoming a widely used measure of quality of life in patients with mood and anxiety disorders. A 16-item short form which corresponds to the general activities section is also available.

Scoring

Items are scored on a 1–5 scale; raw scores for the subscales and the total score are converted to percentages of maximum possible scores where higher scores indicate better quality of life.

Versions

The Q-LES-Q has been translated into over 40 languages.

Additional references

Miller IW, Keitner GI, Schatzberg AF, Klein DN, Thase ME, Rush AJ, Markowitz JC, Schlager DS, Kornstein SG, Davis SM, Harrison WM, Keller MB. The Treatment of Chronic Depression, Part 3: Psychosocial Functioning Before and After Treatment with Sertraline or Imipramine. J Clin Psychiatry 1998; 59(11):608–19.

Russell JM, Koran LM, Rush J, Hirschfeld RM, Harrison W, Friedman ES, Davis S, Keller M. Effect of concurrent anxiety on response to sertraline and imipramine in patients with chronic depression. Depress Anxiety 2001; 13(1):18–27.

Rapaport MH, Endicott J, Clary CM. Posttraumatic stress disorder and quality of life: results across 64 weeks of sertraline treatment. J Clin Psychiatry 2002; 63(1):59–65.

Address for correspondence

Dr. Jean Endicott
Department of Research Assessment and Training
New York State Psychiatric Institute, Unit 123
1051 Riverside Drive
New York, NY 10032, USA
Telephone: 1-212-543-5536
Email: je10@columbia.edu

Quality of Life Enjoyment an Satisfactiond Questionnaire (Q-LES-Q)
Social Relations Sub-scale

	Not at all or never	Rarely	Sometimes	Often or most of the time	Frequently or all the time
During the past week how often have you...					
... enjoyed talking with or being with friends or relatives?	1	2	3	4	5
... looked forward to getting together with friends or relatives?	1	2	3	4	5
... made social plans with friends or relatives for future activities?	1	2	3	4	5
... enjoyed talking with co-workers or neighbors?	1	2	3	4	5
... been patient with others when others were irritating in their actions or words?	1	2	3	4	5
... been interested in the problems of other people?	1	2	3	4	5
... felt affection toward one or more people?	1	2	3	4	5
... gotten along well with other people?	1	2	3	4	5
... joked or laughed with other people?	1	2	3	4	5
... felt you met the needs of friends or relatives?	1	2	3	4	5
... felt your relationships with your friends or relatives were without major problems or conflicts?	1	2	3	4	5

Reproduced from Endicott J, Nee J, Harrison W, Blumenthal R. Psychopharmacol Bull 1993; 29(2):321–6 with permission from Dr Jean Endicott.

Sheehan Disability Scale

Reference: **Sheehan DV. The Anxiety Disease. New York, NY: Charles Scribner's Sons, 1983**

Rating Self-report

Administration time <5 minutes

Main purpose To assess degree of disability

Population Adults

Commentary

The Sheehan Disability Scale is a brief 3-item self-report inventory designed to assess the degree to which symptoms of panic, anxiety, depression or phobia have disrupted the patient's work, social life, and family life. Two additional optional items assess the degree to which symptoms affected productivity in terms of lost or unproductive days. The scale has been used widely in pharmaceutical trials, particularly for panic disorder. For routine clinical practice, it represents a brief, easy to administer measure of disability that is sensitive to change, although it may be of less use in non-working populations.

Scoring

All items are scored on a 0–10 scale, where 0 represents no impairment, 1–3 mild impairment, 4–6 moderate impairment, 7–9 marked impairment, and 10 extreme impairment. The 3 primary items can be summed into a single measure of global impairment (range 0–30). Scores ≥5 on any of the sub-scales are indicative of functional impairment and increased risk of mental disorder.

Versions

The Sheehan Disability Scale has been translated into Danish, Dutch, French, German, Italian, Portuguese, Spanish and Swedish.

Additional references

Sheehan DV, Harnett-Sheehan K, Raj BA. The measurement of disability. Int Clin Psychopharmacol 1996; 11 Suppl 3:89–95.

Leon AC, Olfson M, Portera L, Farber L, Sheehan DV. Assessing psychiatric impairment in primary care with the Sheehan Disability Scale. Int J Psychiatry Med 1997; 27:93–105.

Von Korff M, Katon W, Rutter C, Ludman E, Simon G, Lin E, Bush T. Effect on disability outcomes of a depression relapse prevention program. Psychosom Med 2003; 65(6):938–43.

Address for correspondence

Dr. David V. Sheehan
Institute for Research in Psychiatry
University of South Florida
3515 East Fletcher Avenue
Tampa, FL 33613-4788, USA
Telephone: 1-813-974-4544
Email: dsheehan@hsc.usf.edu

A brief, patient rated, measure of disability and impairment

Please mark ONE circle for each scale

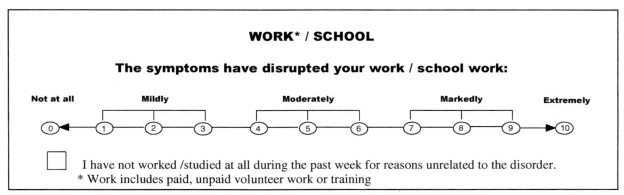

WORK* / SCHOOL

The symptoms have disrupted your work / school work:

I have not worked /studied at all during the past week for reasons unrelated to the disorder.
* Work includes paid, unpaid volunteer work or training

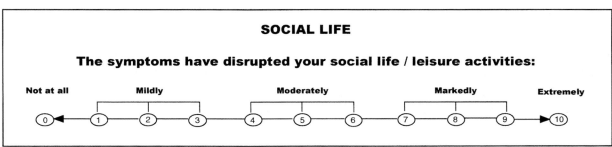

SOCIAL LIFE

The symptoms have disrupted your social life / leisure activities:

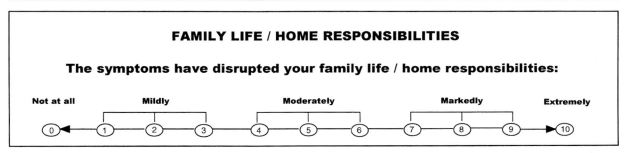

FAMILY LIFE / HOME RESPONSIBILITIES

The symptoms have disrupted your family life / home responsibilities:

Days lost
On how many days in the last week did your symptoms cause you to miss school or work or leave you unable to carry out your normal daily responsibilities? _____

Days underproductive
On how many days in the last week did you feel so impaired by your symptoms, that even though you went to school or work, your productivity was reduced? _____

Short Form McGill Pain Questionnaire (SF-MPQ)

Reference: **Melzack R. The short-form McGill Pain Questionnaire. Pain 1987; 30(2):191–7**

Rating Self-report

Administration time 5 minutes

Main purpose To assess the sensory, affective and other qualitative components of pain

Population Adults, adolescents and older adults

Commentary

The SF-MPQ is a widely used 15-item self-report scale that assesses 11 sensory and 4 affective types of pain. Three pain scores are derived from the sum of the values of the words chosen for sensory, affective and total descriptors. The instrument also includes the Present Pain Intensity (PPI) index of the standard McGill Pain Questionnaire and a visual analogue scale.

Scoring

Items are rated on an intensity scale from 0 (none) through to 3 (severe). Sensory Pain Rating, Affective Pain Rating and Total Pain Rating Indices can be derived, as can a score for the instrument's visual analog scale and indication of overall pain intensity.

Versions

The scale has been translated into: Croatian, Czech, Dutch, French, German, Hebrew, Hungarian, Italian, Polish, Portuguese, Russian, Slovakian, Spanish and Swedish.

Additional reference

Wright KD, Asmundson GJ, McCreary DR. Factorial validity of the short-form McGill pain questionnaire (SF-MPQ). Eur J Pain 2001; 5(3):279–84.

Address for correspondence

Dr. Ronald Melzack
Department of Psychology
McGill University
Montreal, Quebec, Canada
Telephone: 1-514-398-6084
Email: rmelzack@ego.psych.mcgill.ca

Short-Form McGill Pain Questionnaire (SF-MPQ) Form X

A. PLEASE DESCRIBE YOUR PAIN DURING THE LAST WEEK. (√ one box on each line.)

	None	Mild	Moderate	Severe
1. Throbbing	0 ☐	1 ☐	2 ☐	3 ☐
2. Shooting	0 ☐	1 ☐	2 ☐	3 ☐
3. Stabbing	0 ☐	1 ☐	2 ☐	3 ☐
4. Sharp	0 ☐	1 ☐	2 ☐	3 ☐
5. Cramping	0 ☐	1 ☐	2 ☐	3 ☐
6. Gnawing	0 ☐	1 ☐	2 ☐	3 ☐
7. Hot-burning	0 ☐	1 ☐	2 ☐	3 ☐
8. Aching	0 ☐	1 ☐	2 ☐	3 ☐
9. Heavy	0 ☐	1 ☐	2 ☐	3 ☐
10. Tender	0 ☐	1 ☐	2 ☐	3 ☐
11. Splitting	0 ☐	1 ☐	2 ☐	3 ☐
12. Tiring-exhausting	0 ☐	1 ☐	2 ☐	3 ☐
13. Sickening	0 ☐	1 ☐	2 ☐	3 ☐
14. Fearful	0 ☐	1 ☐	2 ☐	3 ☐
15. Punishing-cruel	0 ☐	1 ☐	2 ☐	3 ☐

B. RATE YOUR PAIN DURING THE PAST WEEK

The following line represents pain of increasing intensity from 'no pain' to 'worst possible pain'. Place a slash (|) across the line in the position that best describes your pain **during the past week**.

No
Pain

Worst
possible
pain

Score in mm
(Investigator's use only)

C. PRESENT PAIN INTENSITY

0 ☐ No pain
1 ☐ Mild
2 ☐ Discomforting
3 ☐ Distressing
4 ☐ Horrible
5 ☐ Excruciating

Systematic Assessment for Treatment Emergent Events (SAFTEE)

Reference: **Levine J, Schooler NR. SAFTEE: a technique for the systematic assessment of side effects in clinical trials. Psychopharmacol Bull 1986; 22(2):343–81**

Rating Clinician-rated

Administration time 10–15 minutes

Main purpose To detect and monitor treatment-emergent adverse events

Population Adults and adolescents

Commentary

Developed primarily as a method for eliciting treatment-related adverse events in pharmaceutical trials, the SAFTEE is available in two versions: the SAFTEE-General Inquiry (GI) and SAFTEE-Specific Inquiry (SI). The former uses a general, open-ended interview method to elicit adverse events, and then asks for further information regarding the onset, severity, duration, functional impairment, pattern, etc. of the adverse events identified, regardless of whether they are thought to be drug-related. Results of laboratory and other tests can also be recorded on the form. The SAFTEE-SI involves a full review of systems and makes specific inquiries about symptoms in each area, but may be too time consuming for routine clinical practice. There is debate as to whether the SAFTEE-SI provides additional information over the SAFTEE-GI (see Rabkin et al. 1992 and comment by Levine and Schooler 1992). The SAFTEE-GI can be administered by a wide variety of health professionals, and appears to be a reliable and valid tool for systematically identifying and monitoring treatment-emergent events. The SAFTEE-GI is in the public domain and is reproduced in full here.

Scoring

Summary scores (i.e. number of adverse events experienced) can be calculated, but are rarely used in clinical practice.

Versions

No other versions available.

Additional references

Levine, J. Ascertainment of side effects in psychopharmacologic clinical trials. In: O. Benkert, W. Mair, K. Rickels (eds), Methodology of the Evaluation of Psychotropic Drugs. Psychopharmacology Series 8. New York: Springer-Verlag, pp. 130–135, 1990.

Levine J, Schooler NR. General versus specific inquiry with SAFTEE. J Clin Psychopharmacol 1992; 12(6):448.

Rabkin JG, Markowitz JS, Ocepek-Welikson K, Wager SS. General versus systematic inquiry about emergent clinical events with SAFTEE: implications for clinical research. J Clin Psychopharmacol 1992; 12(1):3–10.

Address for correspondence

Dr. Jerome Levine
Nathan S. Kline Institute for Psychiatric Research
140 Old Orangeburg Road
Orangeburg, NY 10962, USA
Telephone: 1-845-398-5503
Email: levine@nki.rfmh.org

Systematic Assessment for Treatment Emergent Events (SAFTEE)

SAFTEE is designed to collect information on adverse health events occurring during a specified time period of a clinical trial. The SAFTEE-GI form consists of seven components:

- the identifying information on this page;
- Event Terms on pages 2 and 3;
- the examination procedures, printed on the extreme left hand side of pages 4 through 7 and consisting of Opening Remarks, Genenral Inquiry, Closing Inquiry, and Study Specific Events;
- spaces for recording information obtained in the examination, printed next to the examination procedures on pages 4 through 7;
- concluding information printed following the examination procedures on page 4;
- the Laboratory/Physical Findings Record on page 8; and
- the Dosage Record on page 9.

A fuller set of instructions called SAFTEE TIPS is available describing use of this rating system. Briefly, to use the SAFTEE-GI rating system first fill out the identifying information on this page of the booklet. Then go to page 4 and administer the examination beginning with the Opening Remarks (printed on the top left hand side of the page) and continuing with General Inquiry and Closing Inquiry. If an adverse event is detected in the examination, information on that event should be recorded on the form. Suggested queries for eliciting the relevant data are given above each category used to rate the event.

After completing the examination, enter concluding information based upon the examination. This includes the examiner's judgment of patient reliability, any formal diagnoses that can be made, whether an FDA form 1639 is to be filled out, and – if the patient is to be terminated from the trial – the reasons for termination. Dosage information and additional information regarding laboratory and physical findings may be entered at this time or subsequently. The rater should refer to SAFTEE TIPS for complete instructions concerning use of the rating system.

Identifying Information

Patient initials	Age	Sex	Date of assessment
_____	_____	_____	_____

Rater ID _____

Assessment is (select one):
☐ Initial   ☐ Other baseline   ☐ Follow-up   ☐ Final

Assessment is (select one):
☐ Scheduled   ☐ Unscheduled

Assessment interval (i.e. period of time for which events are inquired about):
☐ One week or _____ days

Is the SAFTEE Laboratory/Physical Findings Record to be used with this examination?
☐ Yes   ☐ No

Is the SAFTEE Dosage record to be used with this examination?
☐ Yes   ☐ No

Systematic Assessment for Treatment Emergent Events (SAFTEE)

BEGIN SAFTEE EXAMINATION	To help determine appropriate event category: WHAT KIND OF TROUBLE? CAN YOU TELL ME MORE ABOUT IT? WHERE IS IT? CAN YOU POINT TO IT? IS IT MORE LIKE _____ OR _____? DO YOU HAVE TROUBLE _____?	WHEN DID THIS BEGIN? HAS IT HAPPENED IN THE PAST WEEK? (or specified interval)	HOW LONG DID IT LAST? (only during past week or specified interval)	DID IT HAPPEN MORE THAN ONCE? DID YOU HAVE IT ALL OF THE TIME? PART OF THE TIME?	IS IT A PROBLEM NOW?
_____ _____ Patient ID MM DD YY |___|___| |___|___|					

OPENING REMARKS WE'VE BEEN TALKING ABOUT (name condition being treated). NOW I'D LIKE TO ASK YOU SOME MORE GENERAL QUESTIONS ABOUT YOUR HEALTH. I WANT TO FIND OUT HOW YOU'VE BEEN FEELING IN THE LAST WEEK (or other assessment interval as specified on the first page of the form).	EVENT If event elicited, complete information as requested. (If event previously elicited in General Inquiry, check Prev. Rec. below) * = For event marked with *, record further description in Comments/Description area Lines to record additional events on page 6.	DATE OF ONSET 00.00 = started prior to beginning of this assessment interval MM DD	DURATION IN DAYS (only within current assessment interval) 000 = less than one day	PATTERN IS = isolated IN = intermittent CO = continuous	CURRENT STATUS CO = continuing R = Recovered w/o sequelae RS = Recovered with sequelae I = Indeterminate
GENERAL INQUIRY A. HAVE YOU HAD ANY PHYSICAL OR HEALTH PROBLEMS DURING THE PAST WEEK (or specified interval)? HAVE YOU NOTICED ANY CHANGES IN YOUR PHYSICAL APPEARANCE DURING THE PAST WEEK (or specified assessment interval)? HAVE YOU CUT DOWN ON THE THINGS YOU USUALLY DO BECAUSE OF NOT FEELING WELL PHYSICALLY DURING THE PAST WEEK (or specified assessment interval)? Check if no events elicited ☐	Write in events elicited: If appropriate, use preferred terms listed on pages 2 and 3. 1. _____ 2. _____ 3. _____ 4. _____ 5. _____ 6. _____ 7. _____ 8. _____ 9. _____	__ __ : __ __ __ __ : __ __ __ __ : __ __ __ __ : __ __ __ __ : __ __ __ __ : __ __ __ __ : __ __ __ __ : __ __ __ __ : __ __	__ __	IS IN CO ☐	CO R RS I ☐
IF REQUIRED BY PROTOCOL, GO TO STUDY SPECIFIC EVENTS (NEXT PAGE) OR CONTINUE WITH THE EXAMINATION BELOW. CLOSING INQUIRY B. Observe the patient's appearance and behavior for such problems as skin irritation, weight gain or loss, drowsiness, restlessness, trouble breathing, tremor, rigidity, and other abnormal movements. If the patient fails to mention a problem which has been observed during the examination or which has been reported by staff or family, say: I NOTICE _____ HAS THAT BEEN BOTHERING YOU? Follow up on any problems reported in a previous session that have not been covered in the examination: LAST TIME _____ WAS BOTHERING YOU. ARE YOU STILL HAVING TROUBLE WITH THAT? If no, check assessed & absent Close with (except omit at initial exam.): LASTLY, HAS YOUR MEDICINE CAUSED YOU ANY PROBLEMS DURING THE LAST WEEK (or specified assessment interval) Check if no events elicited ☐	Write in events elicited: If appropriate, use preferred terms listed on pages 2 and 3. assessed & absent 1. _____ ☐ 2. _____ ☐ 3. _____ ☐ 4. _____ ☐ 5. _____ ☐ 6. _____ ☐ 7. _____ ☐ 8. _____ ☐ 9. _____ ☐ 10. _____ ☐ 11. _____ ☐ 12. _____ ☐ 13. _____ ☐	__ __ : __ __ __ __ : __ __ __ __ : __ __ __ __ : __ __ __ __ : __ __ __ __ : __ __ __ __ : __ __ __ __ : __ __ __ __ : __ __ __ __ : __ __ __ __ : __ __ __ __ : __ __ __ __ : __ __	__ __	IS IN CO ☐	CO R RS I ☐

Systematic Assessment for Treatment Emergent Events (SAFTEE)

| HOW BAD IS IT? DOES IT BOTHER YOU A LOT? | DOES IT KEEP YOU FROM DOING THINGS (e.g. eating, sleeping)? HOW HARD IS IT TO (move, stand, stay awake, etc)? If possible observe impairment | IS IT A PROBLEM NOW? IS THIS UNUSUAL FOR YOU? IS THIS SOMETHING YOU'VE ALWAYS HAD? HAS IT CHANGED/GOTTEN WORSE RECENTLY? CAN YOU THINK OF ANYTHING ELSE THAT MIGHT HAVE CAUSED IT? | For Relationship of Drug to Event HAS THERE BEEN ANY CHANGE SINCE WE INCREASED/DECREASED YOUR DOSAGE? (Dose response) HAS THERE BEEN A CHANGE SINCE YOU STOPPED THE DRUG/STARTED IT AGAIN? (De/Rechallenge, not for drug initiation) DOES IT USUALLY HAPPEN RIGHT AFTER YOU TAKE YOUR MEDICINE? (Timing of onset) Relationship may be inferred by examiner if not reported by patient | |

SEVERITY	FUNCTIONAL IMPAIRMENT	POSSIBLE CONTRIBUTORY FACTORS	RELATIONSHIP OF DRUG TO EVENT	ACTION TAKEN (by clinician)
MN = Minimal MI = Mild MO = Moderate S = Severe VS = Very severe	MN = Minimal MI = Mild MO = Moderate S = Severe VS = Very severe	Check as many as apply CD = Current disorder (being treated) II = Intercurrent illness OD = Other disorder (prior) PH = Prior history of event PD = Protocol drug DI = Other drug/drug interaction O = Other (specify) OR N = None apparent	Check as many as apply D = Dose response DR = Dechallenge/rechallenge TO = Timing of onset S = Seen in other patients in this trial K = Known drug effect L = Laboratory data O = Other (specify) OR NA = Not applicable (PD or DI not checked in Contributory Factors column)	N = None IS = Increased surveillance C = Contra-active RX CH = Change dose CC = Contra-active RX plus change dose SU = Suspend RX DC = Discontinue RX O = Other (specify) X = Don't know

STUDY SPECIFIC EVENTS	To help determine appropriate event category: WHAT KIND OF TROUBLE? CAN YOU TELL ME MORE ABOUT IT? WHERE IS IT? CAN YOU POINT TO IT? IS IT MORE LIKE _____ OR _____? DO YOU HAVE TROUBLE _____?	WHEN DID THIS BEGIN? HAS IT HAPPENED IN THE PAST WEEK? (or specified interval)	HOW LONG DID IT LAST? (only during past week or specified interval)	DID IT HAPPEN MORE THAN ONCE? DID YOU HAVE IT ALL OF THE TIME? PART OF THE TIME?	IS IT A PROBLEM NOW?
	EVENT If event elicited, complete information as requested.	**DATE OF ONSET** 00.00 = started prior to beginning of this assessment interval	**DURATION IN DAYS** (only within current assessment interval)	**PATTERN** IS = isolated IN = intermittent CO = continuous	**CURRENT STATUS** CO = continuing R = Recovered w/o sequelae RS = Recovered with sequelae I = Indeterminate
		MM DD	000 = less than one day		

2. (Enter script for Study Specific Events)

	EVENT	DATE OF ONSET	DURATION	PATTERN IS IN CO	CURRENT STATUS CO R RS I
1.	_____	__ __ : __ __	__ __ __	☐ ☐ ☐	☐ ☐ ☐ ☐
2.	_____	__ __ : __ __	__ __ __	☐ ☐ ☐	☐ ☐ ☐ ☐
3.	_____	__ __ : __ __	__ __ __	☐ ☐ ☐	☐ ☐ ☐ ☐
4.	_____	__ __ : __ __	__ __ __	☐ ☐ ☐	☐ ☐ ☐ ☐
5.	_____	__ __ : __ __	__ __ __	☐ ☐ ☐	☐ ☐ ☐ ☐
6.	_____	__ __ : __ __	__ __ __	☐ ☐ ☐	☐ ☐ ☐ ☐
7.	_____	__ __ : __ __	__ __ __	☐ ☐ ☐	☐ ☐ ☐ ☐
8.	_____	__ __ : __ __	__ __ __	☐ ☐ ☐	☐ ☐ ☐ ☐
9.	_____	__ __ : __ __	__ __ __	☐ ☐ ☐	☐ ☐ ☐ ☐
10.	_____	__ __ : __ __	__ __ __	☐ ☐ ☐	☐ ☐ ☐ ☐
11.	_____	__ __ : __ __	__ __ __	☐ ☐ ☐	☐ ☐ ☐ ☐
12.	_____	__ __ : __ __	__ __ __	☐ ☐ ☐	☐ ☐ ☐ ☐
13.	_____	__ __ : __ __	__ __ __	☐ ☐ ☐	☐ ☐ ☐ ☐
14.	_____	__ __ : __ __	__ __ __	☐ ☐ ☐	☐ ☐ ☐ ☐
15.	_____	__ __ : __ __	__ __ __	☐ ☐ ☐	☐ ☐ ☐ ☐
16.	_____	__ __ : __ __	__ __ __	☐ ☐ ☐	☐ ☐ ☐ ☐
17.	_____	__ __ : __ __	__ __ __	☐ ☐ ☐	☐ ☐ ☐ ☐
18.	_____	__ __ : __ __	__ __ __	☐ ☐ ☐	☐ ☐ ☐ ☐

RETURN TO PREVIOUS PAGE FOR CLOSING INQUIRY

WRITE-IN SPACE FOR ADDITIONAL EVENTS	For each write-in: Record query letter, use next number in sequence, and specify.			IS IN CO	CO R RS I
	__ __ _____	__ __ : __ __	__ __ __	☐ ☐ ☐	☐ ☐ ☐ ☐
	__ __ _____	__ __ : __ __	__ __ __	☐ ☐ ☐	☐ ☐ ☐ ☐
	__ __ _____	__ __ : __ __	__ __ __	☐ ☐ ☐	☐ ☐ ☐ ☐
	__ __ _____	__ __ : __ __	__ __ __	☐ ☐ ☐	☐ ☐ ☐ ☐
	__ __ _____	__ __ : __ __	__ __ __	☐ ☐ ☐	☐ ☐ ☐ ☐

Systematic Assessment for Treatment Emergent Events (SAFTEE)

| HOW BAD IS IT? DOES IT BOTHER YOU A LOT? | DOES IT KEEP YOU FROM DOING THINGS (e.g. eating, sleeping)? HOW HARD IS IT TO (move, stand, stay awake, etc)? If possible observe impairment | IS IT A PROBLEM NOW? IS THIS UNUSUAL FOR YOU? IS THIS SOMETHING YOU'VE ALWAYS HAD? HAS IT CHANGED/GOTTEN WORSE RECENTLY? CAN YOU THINK OF ANYTHING ELSE THAT MIGHT HAVE CAUSED IT? | For Relationship of Drug to Event HAS THERE BEEN ANY CHANGE SINCE WE INCREASED/DECREASED YOUR DOSAGE? (Dose response) HAS THERE BEEN A CHANGE SINCE YOU STOPPED THE DRUG/STARTED IT AGAIN? (De/Rechallenge, not for drug initiation) DOES IT USUALLY HAPPEN RIGHT AFTER YOU TAKE YOUR MEDICINE? (Timing of onset) Relationship may be inferred by examiner if not reported by patient | |

SEVERITY	FUNCTIONAL IMPAIRMENT	POSSIBLE CONTRIBUTORY FACTORS	RELATIONSHIP OF DRUG TO EVENT	ACTION TAKEN (by clinician)
MN = Minimal MI = Mild MO = Moderate S = Severe VS = Very severe	MN = Minimal MI = Mild MO = Moderate S = Severe VS = Very severe	Check as many as apply CD = Current disorder (being treated) II = Intercurrent illness OD = Other disorder (prior) PH = Prior history of event PD = Protocol drug DI = Other drug/drug interaction O = Other (specify) 　　OR N = None apparent	Check as many as apply D = Dose response DR = Dechallenge/rechallenge TO = Timing of onset S = Seen in other patients in this trial K = Know drug effect L = Laboratory data O = Other (specify) 　　OR NA = Not applicable (PD or DI not checked in Contributory Factors column)	N = None IS = Increased surveillance C = Contra-active RX CH = Change dose CC = Contra-active RX plus change dose SU = Suspend RX DC = Discontinue RX O = Other (specify) X = Don't know
MN MI MO S VS ☐☐☐☐☐ (×16)	MN MI MO S VS ☐☐☐☐☐ (×16)	CD II OD PH PD DI O or N ☐☐ ☐☐☐☐☐ ☐ (×16)	D DR TO S K L O or NA ☐☐☐☐☐☐☐ ☐ (×16)	N IS C CH CC SU DC O X ☐☐☐☐☐☐☐☐☐ (×16)
MN MI MO S VS ☐☐☐☐☐ (×4)	MN MI MO S VS ☐☐☐☐☐ (×4)	CD II OD PH PD DI O or N ☐☐ ☐☐☐☐☐ ☐ (×4)	D DR TO S K L O or NA ☐☐☐☐☐☐☐ ☐ (×4)	N IS C CH CC SU DC O X ☐☐☐☐☐☐☐☐☐ (×4)

LABORATORY/PHYSICAL FINDINGS RECORD	ASSOCIATION TO EVENT	DATE OF TEST	RESULTS	CLINICAL ABNORMALITY	POSSIBLE CONTRIBUTORY FACTORS	ACTION TAKEN BY CLINICIAN
To be used (1) to record Lab/Physical findings (normal or abnormal) associated with elicited events or (2) to record abnormal Lab/Physical findings not associated with an event.	N = No associated event OR If associated, enter event letter and number		Record value or score using both number and units	Y = Yes N = No X = Uncertain	Enter as many as apply CD = Current disorder (being treated) II = Intercurrent illness OD = Other disorder (prior) PH = Prior history of abnormal test PD = Protocol drug DI = Other drug/drug interaction O = Other (specify) OR N = None apparent	Enter as many as apply N = None R = repeat test IS = Increased surveillance C = Contra-active Rx CH = Change dose SU = Suspend Rx DC = Discontinue Rx O = Other (specify) OR X = Don't know

Use page 19 for comments or to specify where requested.

SPECIFY TEST BELOW — Check if no lab/physical findings are reported ☐

ASSOCIATION TO EVENT: N or event — DATE OF TEST: MM DD

LAB-HEMATOLOGIC

N
☐ or ____ ____
☐ or ____ ____
☐ or ____ ____
☐ or ____ ____

Clinical Abnormality: Y N X
Possible Contributory Factors: CD II OD PH PD DI O or N
Action Taken: N R IS C CH SU DC O or X

LAB-LIVER FUNCTION

N
☐ or ____ ____
☐ or ____ ____
☐ or ____ ____
☐ or ____ ____

Clinical Abnormality: Y N X
Possible Contributory Factors: CD II OD PH PD DI O or N
Action Taken: N R IS C CH SU DC O or X

LAB-KIDNEY

N
☐ or ____ ____
☐ or ____ ____
☐ or ____ ____
☐ or ____ ____

Clinical Abnormality: Y N X
Possible Contributory Factors: CD II OD PH PD DI O or N
Action Taken: N R IS C CH SU DC O or X

LAB-OTHER

N
☐ or ____ ____
☐ or ____ ____
☐ or ____ ____
☐ or ____ ____

Clinical Abnormality: Y N X
Possible Contributory Factors: CD II OD PH PD DI O or N
Action Taken: N R IS C CH SU DC O or X

RADIOLOGIC

N
☐ or ____ ____
☐ or ____ ____
☐ or ____ ____
☐ or ____ ____

Clinical Abnormality: Y N X
Possible Contributory Factors: CD II OD PH PD DI O or N
Action Taken: N R IS C CH SU DC O or X

ELECTRO-PHYSIOLOGIC (e.g. EKG, EEG)

N
☐ or ____ ____
☐ or ____ ____
☐ or ____ ____

Clinical Abnormality: Y N X
Possible Contributory Factors: CD II OD PH PD DI O or N
Action Taken: N R IS C CH SU DC O or X

PHYSICAL FINDINGS (e.g. weight, B.P.)

N
☐ or ____ ____
☐ or ____ ____

Clinical Abnormality: Y N X
Possible Contributory Factors: CD II OD PH PD DI O or N
Action Taken: N R IS C CH SU DC O or X

OTHER (specify)

N
☐ or ____ ____
☐ or ____ ____
☐ or ____ ____
☐ or ____ ____

Clinical Abnormality: Y N X
Possible Contributory Factors: CD II OD PH PD DI O or N
Action Taken: N R IS C CH SU DC O or X

Sickness Impact Profile (SIP)

Reference: **Gilson BS, Gilson JS, Bergner M, Bobbit RA, Kressel S, Pollard WE, Vesselago M. The sickness impact profile. Development of an outcome measure of health care. Am J Public Health 1975; 65(12):1304–10**

Rating Self-report

Administration time >20 minutes

Main purpose To behaviourally assess the impact of sickness

Population Adults

Commentary

The SIP is a 136-item self-report measure of sickness-related dysfunction that assesses 12 primary behavioural domains: sleep and rest, eating, work, home management, recreation and pastimes, ambulation, mobility, body care and movement, social interactions, alertness behaviour, emotional behaviour and communication. The instrument has been used extensively in a wide variety of clinical contexts and patient populations, and research has indicated that the tool has sound psychometric properties and is relatively responsive to change (albeit not over very short time periods). Importantly, the instrument appears to be acceptable to patients, although it may be too time-consuming to administer in some settings.

Scoring

Items are scored in a yes/no fashion, the overall SIP score and sub-scale scores range from 0–100 (percentage of items endorsed yes multiplied by 100). The ambulation, mobility and body care and movement sub-scales can be combined to form a physical domain, and the social interactions, alertness, emotional and communication sub-scales can be combined to form a psychosocial domain; all other sub-scales are independent. The general adult population has a SIP score of approximately 5, an SIP score of >20 indicates the need for substantial daily care, and >30 indicates the need for almost complete care.

Versions

An interviewer-administered form is available, as is a Sickness Impact Profile for Nursing Homes (SIP-NH), a stroke-adapted 30-item version and a short-form (SIP68); the SIP has been translated into Arabic, Chinese, Danish, Dutch, Finnish, French, German, Italian, Norwegian, Portuguese, Russian, Spanish, Swedish, Tamil and Thai.

Additional references

Bergner M, Bobbitt RA, Carter WB, Gilson BS. The Sickness Impact Profile: development and final revision of a health status measure. Med Care 1981; 19(8):787–805.

de Bruin AF, de Witte LP, Stevens F, Diederiks JP. Sickness Impact Profile: the state of the art of a generic functional status measure. Soc Sci Med 1992; 35(8):1003–14.

de Bruin AF, Diederiks JP, de Witte LP, Stevens FC, Philipsen H. The development of a short generic version of the Sickness Impact Profile. J Clin Epidemiol 1994; 47(4):407–18.

Address for correspondence

Medical Outcomes Trust
235 Wyman St., Suite 130
Waltham, MA 02451, USA
Telephone: 781-890-4884
Email: info@outcomes-trust.org
www.outcomes-trust.org

Copyright is held by Johns Hopkins University.

Somatic Symptom Inventory (SSI)

Reference: **Barsky AJ, Wyshak G, Klerman GL. Hypochondriasis. An evaluation of the DSM-III criteria in medical outpatients. Arch Gen Psychiatry 1986; 43(5):493–500**

Rating Self-report

Administration time 7 minutes

Main purpose To assess severity of somatic symptomatology

Population Adults and older adults

Commentary

The original version of the SSI contained 26 items assessing somatic symptoms, body sensations and overall health; a revised 28-item version that also assesses joint and neck pain is now also widely used. The SSI consists of items from both the Symptom Checklist 90's (see page 166) somatization sub-scale and the Minnesota Multiphasic Personality Inventory's hypochondriasis scale. The scale is primarily used as a meure of hypochondriasis and severity of somatic symptoms.

Scoring

Items are scored on a 1 (not at all) to 5 (a great deal) scale, with a total score range of 26–130.

Versions

The scale has been translated into Spanish and French.

Additional references

Barsky AJ, Wyshak G, Klerman GL. Transient hypochondriasis. Arch Gen Psychiat 1990; 47:746–52.

Wyshak G, Barsky AJ, Klerman GL. Comparison of psychiatric screening tests in a general hospital setting using ROC analysis. Med Care 1991; 29:775–85.

Barsky AJ, Wyshak G, Klerman GL. Psychiatric comorbidity in DSM-III-R hypochondriasis. Arch Gen Psychiat 1992; 49:101–8.

Goldstein DJ, Lu Y, Detke MJ, Hudson J, Iyengar S, Demitrack MA. Effects of duloxetine on painful physical symptoms associated with depression. Psychosomatics 2004; 45(1):17–28.

Address for correspondence

Dr. Arthur J. Barsky
Department of Psychiatry
Brigham and Women's Hospital
75 Francis St, Boston, MA 02115, USA
Telephone: 1-617-732-5236
Email: abarsky@partners.org

Somatic Symptom Inventory (SSI)

Below is a list of symptoms. For each one, please circle the number indicating how much it has bothered you over the past **6 months.**

1 = Not at all
2 = A little bit
3 = Moderately
4 = Quite a bit
5 = A great deal

1)	Nausea or vomiting	1	2	3	4	5
2)	Soreness in your muscles	1	2	3	4	5
3)	Pains or cramps in your abdomen	1	2	3	4	5
4)	Feeling faint or dizzy	1	2	3	4	5
5)	Trouble with your vision	1	2	3	4	5
6)	Your muscles twitching or jumping	1	2	3	4	5
7)	Feeling fatigued, weak, or tired all over	1	2	3	4	5
8)	A fullness in your head or nose	1	2	3	4	5
9)	Pains in your lower back	1	2	3	4	5
10)	Constipation	1	2	3	4	5
11)	Trouble catching your breath	1	2	3	4	5
12)	Hot or cold spells	1	2	3	4	5
13)	A ringing or buzzing in your ears	1	2	3	4	5
14)	Pains in your heart or chest	1	2	3	4	5
15)	Difficulty keeping your balance while walking	1	2	3	4	5
16)	Indigestion, upset stomach, or acid stomach	1	2	3	4	5
17)	The feeling that you are not in as good physical health as most of your friends	1	2	3	4	5
18)	Numbness, tingling, or burning in parts of your body	1	2	3	4	5
19)	Headaches	1	2	3	4	5
20)	A lump in your throat	1	2	3	4	5
21)	Feeling weak in parts of your body	1	2	3	4	5
22)	Not feeling well most of the time in the past few years	1	2	3	4	5
23)	Heavy feelings in your arms or legs	1	2	3	4	5
24)	Your heart pounding, turning over, or missing a beat	1	2	3	4	5
25)	Your hands and feet not feeling warm enough	1	2	3	4	5
26)	The sense that your hearing is not as good as it used to be	1	2	3	4	5

Reproduced from Barsky AJ, Wyshak G, Klerman GL. Arch Gen Psychiatry 1986; 43(5):493–500. © Arthur J Barsky 2003.

Symptom Checklist-90–Revised (SCL-90-R)

Reference: **Derogatis LR. Symptom Checklist 90-R: Administration, Scoring and Procedures Manual. 1983. Baltimore, MD, Clinical Psychometric Research**

Rating Self-report

Administration time 15 minutes

Main purpose To screen for global psychopathology

Population Adults and adolescents

Commentary

The SCL-90-R is a 90-item self-report inventory designed to screen for psychological distress and global psychopathology over the past week. The scale contains 9 symptom domains: depression, anxiety, hostility, interpersonal sensitivity, obsessive-compulsive, somatization, paranoid ideation, phobic anxiety and psychoticism. It also yields 3 global indices: the global severity index, the positive symptom distress index and the positive symptom total. As a screening tool, the instrument has been widely used and holds clinical utility, but the depression and anxiety symptom scales are not particularly well validated, and the majority of the instrument's items assess other constructs. The SCL-90-R represents a useful adjunctive measure of global psychological distress, but is not recommended for use in isolation to assess severity of, or change in, symptoms of depression or anxiety.

Scoring

Items are scored either by hand or computer on a 0 (not at all) to 4 (extremely) scale, with a total possible score of 360. The global severity index represents the mean of all items (the number of items per sub-scale varies). One study has suggested a cut-off point of 0.57 on the global severity index to differentiate 'functional' and 'dysfunctional' populations (Schauenburg and Strack 1999).

Versions

A computerized version of the SCL-90-R is available, and the scale has been translated into Arabic, Chinese, Danish, Dutch, French, French for Canada, German, Hebrew, Italian, Japanese, Korean, Norwegian, Portuguese, Spanish, Swedish and Vietnamese.

Additional references

Schauenburg H, Strack M. Measuring psychotherapeutic change with the symptom checklist SCL 90 R. Psychother Psychosom 1999; 68(4):199–206.

Schmitz N, Kruse J, Heckrath C, Alberti L, Tress W. Diagnosing mental disorders in primary care: the General Health Questionnaire (GHQ) and the Symptom Check List (SCL-90-R) as screening instruments. Soc Psychiatry Psychiatr Epidemiol 1999; 34(7):360–6.

Address for correspondence

Multi-Health Systems Inc.
P.O. Box 950
North Tonawanda, NY 14120-0950, USA
Telephone: 1-800-456-3003 in the US
or 1-416-492-2627 international
Email: customerservice@mhs.com
Website: www.mhs.com

Chapter 5

Special populations

Depression and anxiety are more difficult to assess and diagnose in special populations, such as child and adolescent and geriatric age groups, in the medically ill and in different cultural groups. The symptoms of mood and anxiety disorders are often quite different in children. When depressed, children (and adolescents) often become irritable, withdraw from others, or stop playing rather than showing sad mood or loss of pleasure. Instead of weight loss, they may not reach expected weight for age. Instead of subjective anxiety, children may cry, throw temper tantrums, freeze up or avoid interactions with unfamiliar people. Children may also not recognize that symptoms are excessive or unreasonable, for example, in obsessions and compulsions or in social anxiety. In post traumatic stress disorder, children may respond to trauma with disorganized or agitated behaviour instead of fearfulness. They may also re-enact the trauma or themes of the trauma in play, or have frightening dreams without recollection of content. In social anxiety disorder, children must show symptoms with peers and not just in interactions with adults.

In geriatric and some cross-cultural populations, somatic presentations are often more prominent. In older adults, depression is often intertwined with grief and bereavement, as many symptoms are common between them. Symptoms that can help distinguish major depression from bereavement include marked psychomotor retardation, suicidal ideation, feelings of worthlessness and pathological guilt (especially about things unrelated to the deceased) in the former. Older adults are also prone to delusional guilt, for example, nihilistic delusions and delusions of poverty.

In the medically ill, symptoms of the medical illness or the side effects of medications used to treat the disorder can mask or mimic the vegetative symptoms of depression. Scales designed to identify depression in people with comorbid medical illnesses often focus on cognitive symptoms rather than vegetative ones, which are more likely to be confused with the symptoms of the medical illness.

Beck Depression Inventory – Fast Screen for Medical Patients (BDI-FS)

Reference: **Beck AT, Steer RA, Brown GK. BDI-FastScreen for Medical Patients Manual. 2000. San Antonio, TX, The Psychological Corporation**

Rating Self-report

Administration time <5 minutes

Main purpose To screen for depression in medical patients

Population Adults and adolescents

Commentary

The BDI-FS is a 7-item self-report questionnaire specifically designed to evaluate depression in patients whose behavioral and somatic symptoms may be attributable to biological, medical, alcohol and/or substance use problems. Focusing solely upon the cognitive and affective symptoms of depression, it provides a rapid method for screening for depression in medical patients. Research has indicated that it is also an effective screening tool in geriatric patients.

Scoring

No details available.

Versions

No other versions are available at present.

Additional references

Scheinthal SM, Steer RA, Giffin L, Beck AT. Evaluating geriatric medical outpatients with the Beck Depression Inventory-Fastscreen for medical patients. Aging Ment Health 2001; 5(2):143–8.

Benedict RH, Fishman I, McClellan MM, Bakshi R, Weinstock-Guttman B. Validity of the Beck Depression Inventory-Fast Screen in multiple sclerosis. Mult Scler 2003; 9(4):393–6.

Address for correspondence

Harcourt Assessment, Inc.
19500 Bulverde Road
San Antonio, TX 78259, USA
Telephone: 1-800-2111-8378
Website: www.HarcourtAssessment.com

Calgary Depression Scale for Schizophrenia (CDSS)

Reference: **Addington D, Addington J, Maticka-Tyndale E. Assessing depression in schizophrenia: the Calgary Depression Scale. Br J Psychiatry Suppl 1993; Dec(22):39–44**

Rating Clinician-rated

Administration time 20 minutes

Main purpose To assess depressive symptoms in patients with schizophrenia

Population Adults and adolescents diagnosed with schizophrenia

Commentary

The CDSS is a 9-item clinician-rated scale developed to assess symptoms of major depressive disorder over the past two weeks in patients with schizophrenia. Compared with the Hamilton Depression Rating Scale or HDRS (see page 28), the CDSS has fewer factors and less overlap with positive and negative symptoms of schizophrenia (Addington et al., 1996). This suggests that it is a more specific measure of level of depression than the HDRS for individuals with schizophrenia. Note that the scale is designed for use by clinicians with experience in this patient population. The scale developers suggest that new raters should optimize inter-rater reliability by collaborating with another clinician experienced in the use of structured assessment instruments, and that experienced raters should develop adequate inter-rater reliability within 5 practice interviews. The CDSS appears to be a reliable and valid measure of depressive symptoms in patients with schizophrenia that is appropriate for use both as a screening instrument and as an outcome measure.

Scoring

Items are scored on a 0 (absent) to 3 (severe) basis; detailed anchor points are provided for each item. A total score (range 0–27) is calculated by summing all items. A score of ≥5 is typically used to identify patients with comorbid major depression.

Versions

The CDSS is available in a wide range of languages including: Czech, Danish, Dutch, Finnish, French, German, Greek, Hebrew, Hungarian, Italian, Japanese, Korean, Mandarin, Norwegian, Polish, Portuguese, Romanian, Russian, Spanish, Swedish, Togalog and Turkish.

Additional references

Addington D, Addington J, Atkinson M. A psychometric comparison of the Calgary Depression Scale for Schizophrenia and the Hamilton Depression Rating Scale. Schizophr Res 1996; 19(2–3):205–12.

Kontaxakis VP, Havaki-Kontaxaki BJ, Stamouli SS, Margariti MM, Collias CT, Christodoulou GN. Comparison of four scales measuring depression in schizophrenic inpatients. Eur Psychiatry 2000; 15(4):274–7.

Reine G, Lancon C, Di Tucci S, Sapin C, Auquier P. Depression and subjective quality of life in chronic phase schizophrenic patients. Acta Psychiatr Scand 2003; 108(4):297–303.

Address for correspondence

Dr. Donald Addington
Department of Psychiatry
Foothills Hospital, 1403 – 29th Street NW
Calgary, Alberta T2N 2T9, Canada
Telephone: 1-403-944-1296
Email: addingto@ucalgary.ca
Website: www.ucalgary.ca/cdss

Calgary Depression Scale for Schizophrenia (CDSS)

Interviewer: Ask the first question as written. Use follow up probes or qualifiers at your discretion. Time frame refers to last two weeks unless stipulated. **N.B.** The last item, #9, is based on observations of the entire interview.

1. DEPRESSION: How would you describe your mood over the last two weeks? Do you keep reasonably cheerful or have you been very depressed or low spirited recently? In the last two weeks how often have you (own words) every day? All day?

0	Absent	
1	Mild	Expresses some sadness or discouragement on questioning.
2	Moderate	Distinct depressed mood persisting up to half the time over last 2 weeks: present daily.
3	Severe	Markedly depressed mood persisting daily over half the time interfering with normal motor and social functioning.

2. HOPELESSNESS: How do you see the future for yourself? Can you see any future? – or has life seemed quite hopeless? Have you given up or does there still seem some reason for trying?

0	Absent	
1	Mild	Has at times felt hopeless over the last two weeks but still has some degree of hope for the future.
2	Moderate	Persistent, moderate sense of hopelessness over last week. Can be persuaded to acknowledge possibility of things being better.
3	Severe	Persisting and distressing sense of hopelessness.

3. SELF DEPRECIATION: What is your opinion of your self compared to other people? Do you feel better, not as good, or about the same as other? Do you feel inferior or even worthless?

0	Absent	
1	Mild	Some inferiority; not amounting to feeling of worthlessness.
2	Moderate	Subject feels worthless, but less than 50% of the time.
3	Severe	Subject feels worthless more than 50% of the time. May be challenged to acknowledge otherwise.

4. GUILTY IDEAS OF REFERENCE: Do you have the feeling that you are being blamed for something or even wrongly accused? What about? (Do not include justifiable blame or accusation. Exclude delusions of guilt.)

0	Absent	
1	Mild	Subject feels blamed but not accused less than 50% of the time.
2	Moderate	Persisting sense of being blamed, and/or occasional sense of being accused.
3	Severe	Persistent sense of being accused. When challenged, acknowledges that it is not so.

5. PATHOLOGICAL GUILT: Do you tend to blame yourself for little things you may have done in the past? Do you think that you deserve to be so concerned about this?

0	Absent	
1	Mild	Subject sometimes feels over guilty about some minor peccadillo, but less than 50% of time.
2	Moderate	Subject usually (over 50% of time) feels guilty about past actions the significance of which he exaggerates.
3	Severe	Subject usually feels s/he is to blame for everything that has gone wrong, even when not his/her fault.

6. MORNING DEPRESSION: When you have felt depressed over the last 2 weeks have you noticed the depression being worse at any particular time of day?

0	Absent	No depression.
1	Mild	Depression present but no diurnal variation.
2	Moderate	Depression spontaneously mentioned to be worse in a.m.
3	Severe	Depression markedly worse in a.m., with impaired functioning which improves in p.m.

7. EARLY WAKENING: Do you wake earlier in the morning than is normal for you? How many times a week does this happen?

0	Absent	No early wakening.
1	Mild	Occasionally wakes (up to twice weekly) 1 hour or more before normal time to wake or alarm time.
2	Moderate	Often wakes early (up to 5 times weekly) 1 hour or more before normal time to wake or alarm.
3	Severe	Daily wakes 1 hour or more before normal time.

8. SUICIDE: Have you felt that life wasn't worth living? Did you ever feel like ending it all? What did you think you might do? Did you actually try?

0	Absent	
1	Mild	Frequent thoughts of being better off dead, or occasional thoughts of suicide.
2	Moderate	Deliberately considered suicide with a plan, but made no attempt.
3	Severe	Suicidal attempt apparently designed to end in death (i.e.: accidental discovery of inefficient means).

9. OBSERVED DEPRESSION: Based on interviewer's observations during the entire interview. The question 'Do you feel like crying?' used at appropriate points in the interview, may elicit information useful to this observation.

0	Absent	
1	Mild	Subject appears sad and mournful even during parts of the interview, involving affectively neutral discussion.
2	Moderate	Subject appears sad and mournful throughout the interview, with gloomy monotonous voice and is tearful or close to tears at times.
3	Severe	Subject chokes on distressing topics, frequently sighs deeply and cries openly, or is persistently in a state of frozen misery if examiner is sure that this is present.

Reproduced from Addington D, Addington J, Maticka-Tyndale E. Br J Psychiatry Suppl 1993; Dec(22):39–44. © Donald Addington 2004.

Children's Depression Inventory (CDI)

Reference: **Kovacs M. Children's Depression Inventory Manual. 1992. North Tonawanda, NY, Multi-Health Systems**

Rating Self-report

Administration time 10–15 minutes

Main purpose To assess depressive symptomatology in children and adolescents

Population Children and adolescents aged 7–17 years

Commentary

The CDI is a widely used 27-item self-report instrument designed to assess symptoms of depression in children and adolescents. The scale, modeled after the Beck Depression Inventory (see page 10), measures symptoms thought to be particularly characteristic of childhood depression such as low mood, poor self-evaluation, and interpersonal problems. The instrument yields 5 sub-scales: negative mood, interpersonal problems, ineffectiveness, anhedonia, and negative self-esteem. The CDI has been found to correlate with other measures of childhood depression, such as the Reynolds Adolescent Depression Scale-2 (see page 185). Numerous studies have demonstrated that children with depression score significantly higher on the scale than non-depressed control subjects. There is some evidence that the instrument is sensitive to change, although the scale has been used most widely as a screening tool for depression in epidemiological studies. A 10-item version of the CDI has also been developed as a more concise screening measure.

Scoring

Items are scored on a 0 (absence of symptom) through to 2 (definite symptom) scale. A total score (range 0–54, where higher scores indicate greater depression severity) is calculated by summing all items; sub-scale scores are derived by totaling the appropriate items. Scores are converted to standardized scores based on age range (7–12 or 13–17 years) and gender. The manual provides the following guidelines for interpreting scores: <30, very much below average, 30–34, much below average, 35–39, below average, 40–44, slightly below average, 45–55, average, 56–60, slightly above average, 61–65, above average, 66–70, much above average, >70, very much above average.

Versions

The scale has been translated into: Arabic, Bulgarian, French-Canadian, French, German, Hebrew, Hungarian, Italian, Portuguese and Spanish. A computer-administered version is available from Multi-Health Systems Inc.

Additional references

Kovacs M. The Children's Depression, Inventory (CDI). Psychopharmacol Bull 1985; 21(4):995–8.

Smucker MR, Craighead WE, Craighead LW, Green BJ. Normative and reliability data for the Children's Depression Inventory. J Abnorm Child Psychol 1986; 14(1):25–39.

Address for correspondence

Multi-Health Systems Inc.
P.O. Box 950
North Tonawanda, NY 14120-0950, USA
Telephone: 1-800-456-3003 in the US
or 1-416-492-2627 international
Email: customerservice@mhs.com
Website: www.mhs.com

Children's Depression Rating Scale–Revised (CDRS-R)

Reference: **Poznanski EO, Mokros HB. Children's Depression Rating Scale–Revised: Manual. 1996. Los Angeles, CA, Western Psychological Services**

Rating Clinician-rated

Administration time 15–20 minutes

Main purpose To screen for and diagnose depression in children, and assess treatment response

Population Children aged 6–12 years

Commentary

The CDRS-R is a 17-item clinician-rated instrument modeled after the HDRS (see page 28) that assesses 17 symptom areas, including those that serve as DSM-IV criteria for a diagnosis of depression. Fourteen of the scale's items are based on child report, with a further 3 items being based upon the child's non-verbal behaviour. The clinician is required to determine a 'Best Description of the Child' rating based on all available information from multiple informants. The CDRS-R has been used successfully in both pediatric and adolescent populations. The scale shows reasonable psychometric properties (good inter-rater and test–retest reliability and internal consistency, and moderate to good validity) and has been used in a variety of clinical trials, although it may prove too unwieldy for use in routine clinical practice.

Scoring

Items are rated either on 7-point or 5-point scales, with detailed anchor points provided. The scale yields a raw summary score (range 17–113) from which a standardized score is calculated. T scores between 55 and 64 indicate a need for further evaluation; scores ≥65 indicate likely depressive disorder.

Versions

No other versions are currently available.

Additional references

Poznanski EO, Cook SC, Carroll BJ. A depression rating scale for children. Pediatrics 1979; 64(4):442–50.

Wagner KD, Ambrosini P, Rynn M, Wohlberg C, Yang R, Greenbaum MS, Childress A, Donnelly C, Deas D; Sertraline Pediatric Depression Study Group. Efficacy of sertraline in the treatment of children and adolescents with major depressive disorder: two randomized controlled trials. JAMA 2003; 290(8):1033–41.

Address for correspondence

Western Psychological Services
12031 Wilshire Blvd.
Los Angeles, CA 90025-1251, USA
Telephone: 1-800-648-8857 (U.S. and Canada only)
International: 1-310-478-2061
Email: custsvc@wpspublish.com
Website: www.wpspublish.com

1 Difficulty having fun

Interest and activities realistically appropriate for age, personality and social environment. No appreciable change from usual behavior during at least the past 2 weeks. Any feelings of boredom are seen as transient.

Describes some activities as enjoyable that are realistically available several times a week but not on a daily basis. Shows interest but not enthusiasm.

Is easily bored. Complains of 'nothing to do' as characteristic of daily experience. Participates in structured activities with a 'going through the motions' attitude. May express interest primarily in activities that are (realistically) unavailable on a daily or weekly basis.

Has no initiative to become involved in any activities. Describes himself/herself as primarily passive. Watches others play or watches TV but shows little interest. Requires coaxing and/or pushing to get involved in activity. Shows no enthusiasm or real interest. Has difficulty naming activities.

2 Depressed Feelings

Occasional feelings of unhappiness that quickly disappear.

Describes sustained periods of unhappiness that appear excessive for events described.

Feels unhappy most of the time without a major precipitating cause

Feels unhappy all of the time; characterized by a sense of psychic pain (e.g. 'I can't stand it')

3 Suicidal ideation

Understands the word *suicide*, but does not apply the term to himself/herself

Sharp denial of suicidal thoughts

Has thoughts about suicide, or of hurting himself/herself (if he/she does not understand the concept of suicide), usually when angry

Has recurrent thoughts of suicide

Has made a suicide attempt within the last month or is actively suicidal

4 Low self-esteem

Describes himself/herself in primarily positive terms

Describes one important or prominent area where he/she feels there is a deficit

Describes himself/herself in predominantly negative terms or gives bland answers to questions asked

Refers to himself/herself in derogatory terms. Reports that other children frequently refer to him/her by using derogratory nicknames. Puts himself/herself down.

Cornell Scale for Depression in Dementia (CSDD)

Reference: **Alexopoulos GS, Abrams RC, Young RC, Shamoian CA. Cornell Scale for Depression in Dementia. Biol Psychiatry 1988; 23(3):271–84**

Rating Clinician-rated

Administration time 30 minutes (20 minutes for the caregiver interview and 10 minutes for the patient interview)

Main purpose To assess depressive symptomatology in people with dementia

Population Patients with dementia

Commentary

The CSDD is a 19-item instrument designed to assess symptoms of depression over the past week in patients diagnosed with dementia. The scale is clinician-administered and uses information from interviews with both the patient and a nursing staff member or other knowledgeable caregiver. Although there is no published manual for the scale, administration instructions are provided in Alexopoulos et al. (1988). The CSDD shows good psychometric properties; scores on the scale are well-correlated with scores on the Hamilton Depression Rating Scale (see page 28), and the instrument is sensitive to change. The scale is in the public domain and is reproduced in full here.

Scoring

Items are scored a 3-point scale ranging from 0 (absent) through to 2 (severe), or the rater can select an 'unable to evaluate' response. Total score range for the instrument is 0 to 38, with higher scores indicating greater severity of depression. A cut-off score of ≥8 has been used to identify depression in patients with dementia (this should be lowered to ≥7 in patients without dementia).

Versions

The scale has been translated into most European languages, Chinese, Korean and Japanese.

Additional references

Vida S, Des Rosiers P, Carrier L, Gauthier S. Depression in Alzheimer's disease: receiver operating characteristic analysis of the Cornell Scale for Depression in Dementia and the Hamilton Depression Scale. J Geriatr Psychiatry Neurol 1994; 7(3):159–62.

Cohen CI, Hyland K, Kimhy D. The utility of mandatory depression screening of dementia patients in nursing homes. Am J Psychiatry 2003; 160(11):2012–17.

Address for correspondence

Dr. George S. Alexopoulos
Weill Medical College of Cornell University
Weill-Cornell Institute of Geriatric Psychiatry
21 Bloomingdale Road
White Plains, NY 10605, USA
Telephone: 1-914-997-5767
Email: gsalexop@med.cornell.edu

Cornell Scale for Depression in Dementia (CSDD)

INTERVIEW WITH THE INFORMANT

Who qualifies as an Informant? Informants should know and have frequent contact with the patient. Reliable informants can include nursing staff for patients in the hospital and nursing homes or a family member for outpatients.

The informant interview should be conducted first. The interviewer should ask about any change in symptoms of depression over the prior week. The rater should complete each item on the scale. The rater can expand on the descriptions of the symptoms in order to help the informant understand each item.

Interview Instructions: I am going to ask you questions about how your relative has been feeling **during the past week**. I am interested in changes you have noticed and the duration of these changes.

A. Mood Related Signs

1. **Anxiety:** *(anxious expression, ruminations, worrying)* Has your relative been feeling anxious this past week? Has s/he been worrying about things s/he may not ordinarily worry about, or ruminating over things that may not be that important? Has your relative had an anxious, tense, distressed or apprehensive expression?

2. **Sadness:** *(sad expression, sad voice, tearfulness)* Has your relative been feeling down, sad, or blue this past week? Has s/he been crying at all? How many days out of the past week has s/he been feeling like this? For how long each day?

3. **Lack of reactivity to pleasant events:** If a pleasant event were to occur today (i.e., going out with spouse, friends, seeing grandchildren), would your relative be able to enjoy it fully, or might his/her mood get in the way of his/her interest in the event or activity? Does your relative's mood affect any of the following:
   - his/her ability to enjoy activities that used to give him/her pleasure?
   - his/her surroundings?
   - his/her feelings for family and friends?

4. **Irritability:** *(easily annoyed, short tempered)* Has your relative felt short-tempered or easily annoyed this past week? Has s/he been feeling irritable, impatient, or angry this week?

B. Behavioral Disturbance

5. **Agitation:** *(restlessness, handwringing, hairpulling)* Has your relative been so fidgety or restless this past week that s/he was unable to sit still for at least an hour? Was your relative so physically agitated that you or others noticed it? Agitation may include such behaviors as playing with one's hands, hair, hand-wringing, hair-pulling, and/or lip-biting: have you observed any such behavior in your relative during the past week?

6. **Retardation:** *(slow movements, slow speech, slow reactions)* Has your relative been talking or moving more slowly than is normal for him/her? This may include:
   - slowness of thoughts and speech
   - delayed response to your questions
   - decreased motor activity and/or reactions.

7. **Multiple physical complaints:** In the past week, has your relative had any of the following physical symptoms? (in excess of what is normal for him/her):
   - indigestion?
   - constipation?
   - diarrhea?
   - stomach cramps?
   - belching?
   - joint pain?
   - backaches?
   - muscles aches?
   - frequent urination?
   - sweating?
   - headaches?
   - heart palpitations?
   - hyperventilation (shortness of breath)?

If you have observed any of these physical symptoms, how much have these things been bothering your relative? How severe have the symptoms gotten? How often have they occurred in the past week?
Rating guideline: Do not rate symptoms that are side effects from medications or those symptoms that are only related to gastrointestinal ailments.

8. **Acute loss of interest:** *(less involved in usual activities)* How has your relative been spending his/her time this past week (not including work and chores)? Has your relative felt interested in his/her usual activities and hobbies? Has your relative spent any *less* time engaging in these activities?

   If s/he is **not** as interested, or has not been that engaged in activities during the past week: Has your relative had to push him/herself to do the things s/he normally enjoys? Has your relative *stopped* doing anything s/he used to do? Can s/he look forward to anything or has s/he lost interest in many of the hobbies from which s/he used to derive pleasure?
   Rating guideline: Ratings of this item should be based on loss of interest during the past week. This item should be rated 0 if the loss of interest is long-standing (longer than 1 month) and there has been no worsening during the past month. This item should be rated 0 if the patient has not been engaged in activities because of physical illness or disability, or if the patient has persistent apathy associated with dementia.

C. Physical Signs

9. **Appetite loss:** *(eating less than usual)* How has your relative's appetite been this past week compared to normal? Has it decreased at all? Has your relative felt less hungry or had to remind him/herself to eat? Have others had to urge or force him/her to eat?
   Rating guideline: Rate 1 if there is appetite loss but still s/he is eating on his/her own. Rate 2 if eats only with others' encouragement or urging.

10. **Weight loss:** Has your relative lost any weight in the past month that s/he has not meant to or been trying to lose? (If not sure: are your relative's clothes any looser on him/her?) If weight loss is associated with present illness (i.e., not due to diet or exercise): how many pounds has s/he lost?
    Rating guideline: Rate 2 if weight loss is greater than 5 lbs. in past month.

11. **Lack of energy:** *(fatigues easily, unable to sustain activities - score only if change occurred acutely, or in less than one month)* How has your relative's energy been this past week compared to normal? Has s/he been tired all the time? Has s/he asked to take naps because of fatigue? This week, has your relative had any of the following symptoms due to lack of energy only (**not** due to physical problems):
    - heaviness in limbs, back, or head?
    - felt like s/he is dragging through the day?

    Has your relative been fatigued more easily this week?
    Rating guideline: Ratings of this item should be based on lack of energy during the week prior to the interview. This item should be rated 0 if the lack of energy is long-standing (longer than 1 month) and there has been no worsening during the past month.

D. Cyclic Functions

12. **Diurnal variation of mood:** *(symptoms worse in the morning)* Regarding your relative's mood (his/her feelings and symptoms of depression), is there any part of the day in which s/he usually feels better or worse? (or does it not make any difference, or vary according to the day or situation?)

If **yes** to a difference in mood during the day: Is your relative's depression worse in the morning or the evening?
If worse in the morning: Is this a mild or a very noticeable difference?

    Rating guideline: Diurnal variation of mood is only rated for symptoms that are worse in the morning. Variation of mood in the evening can be related to sundowning in patients with dementia and should not be rated.

13. **Difficulty falling asleep:** *(later than usual for this individual)* Has your relative had any trouble falling asleep this past week? Does it take him/her longer than usual to fall asleep once s/he gets into bed (i.e., more than 30 min)?

    Rating guideline: Rate 1 if patient only had trouble falling asleep a few nights in the past week. Rate 2 if s/he has had difficulty falling asleep every night this past week.

14. **Multiple awakenings during sleep:** Has your relative been waking up in the middle of the night this past week? How long is s/he awake?
If **yes**: does s/he get out of bed? Is this just to go to the bathroom and then s/he goes back to sleep?

    Rating guideline: Do not rate if waking is only to go to the bathroom and then is able to fall right back asleep. Rate 1 if sleep has only been restless and disturbed occasionally in the past week, and has not gotten out of bed (besides going to the bathroom). Rate 2 if s/he gets out of bed in the middle of the night (for reasons other than voiding), and/or has been waking up every night in the past week.

15. **Early morning awakenings:** *(earlier than usual for this individual)* Has your relative been waking up any earlier this week than s/he normally does (without an alarm clock or someone waking him/her up)?
If **yes**: how much earlier is s/he waking up than is normal for him/her? Does your relative get out of bed when s/he wakes up early, or does s/he stay in bed and/or go back to sleep?

    Rating guideline: Rate 1 if s/he wakes up on his/her own but then goes back to sleep. Rate 2 if s/he wakes earlier than usual and then gets out of bed for the day (i.e., s/he cannot fall back asleep).

E. Ideational Disturbance

16. **Suicide:** *(feels life is not worth living, has suicidal wishes, or makes suicide attempt)* During the past week, has your relative had any thoughts that life is not worth living or that s/he would be better off dead? Has s/he had any thoughts of hurting or even killing him/herself?

    Rating guideline: Rate 1 for passive suicidal ideation (i.e., feels life isn't worth living but has no plan). Rate 2 for active suicidal wishes, and/or any recent suicide attempts, gestures, or plans. History of suicide attempt without current passive or active suicidal ideation is not scored.

17. **Self-depreciation:** *(self-blame, poor self-esteem, feelings of failure)* How has your relative been feeling about him/herself this past week? Has s/he been feeling especially critical of him/herself, feeling that s/he has done things wrong or let others down? Has s/he been feeling guilty about anything s/he has or has not done? Has s/he been comparing him/herself to others, or feeling worthless, or like a failure? Has s/he described him/herself as "no good" or "inferior"?

    Rating guideline: Rate 1 for loss of self-esteem or self-reproach. Rate 2 for feelings of failure, or statements that s/he is "worthless", "inferior", or "no good".

18. **Pessimism:** *(anticipation of the worst)* Has your relative felt pessimistic or discouraged about his/her future this past week? Can your relative see his/her situation improving? Can your relative be reassured by others that things will be okay or that his/her situation will improve?

    Rating guideline: Rate 1 if s/he feels pessimistic, but can be reassured by self or others. Rate 2 if feels hopeless and cannot be reassured that his/her future will be okay.

19. **Mood congruent delusions:** *(delusions of poverty, illness, or loss)* Has your relative been having ideas that others may find strange? Does your relative think his/her present illness is a punishment, or that s/he has brought it on him/herself in some irrational way? Does your relative think s/he has less money or material possessions than s/he really does?

Reproduced from Alexopoulos GS, Abrams RC, Young RC, Shamoian CA. Biol Psychiatry 1988; 23(3):271–84 with permission from Elsevier.

Edinburgh Postnatal Depression Scale (EPDS)

Reference: **Cox JL, Holden JM. Perinatal Mental Health: a Guide to the Edinburgh Postnatal Depression Scale. 2003. London, UK, Gaskell (Royal College of Psychiatrists)**

Rating Self-report

Administration time <5 minutes

Main purpose To screen for postnatal depression

Population Women who have recently given birth

Commentary

The EPDS is a 10-item self-report questionnaire designed to identify women with postnatal depression. The scale appears to have excellent face validity, and has been used extensively to screen for depression in new mothers, both in English speaking and non-English speaking communities. Although it is recommended that the EPDS be used at 6–8 weeks postpartum, there is some evidence that the scale can be used in the immediate postpartum period to identify at-risk mothers. The instrument has also been used to assess mood in new fathers. Although the EPDS may be better at identifying depressed postnatal women with anhedonic and anxious symptomatology rather than those whose depression presents mainly with psychomotor retardation (Guedeney et al., 2000), it represents a rapid, internationally accepted screening tool for postnatal depression.

Scoring

Items are scored on a 0 to 3 basis (the scale uses some reverse scoring) yielding a total score range of 0–30. The authors suggest a cut-off score of 12 for further evaluation.

Versions

The EPDS has been translated into numerous languages, including: Arabic, Chinese (Mandarin), Czech, Dutch, French, German, Greek, Hebrew, Hindi, Icelandic, Italian, Japanese, Maltese, Norwegian, Portuguese, Punjabi, Slovenian, Spanish, Swedish, Urdu and Vietnamese. A computerized version is also available.

Additional references

Cox JL, Holden JM, Sagovsky R. Detection of postnatal depression. Development of the 10-item Edinburgh Postnatal Depression Scale. Br J Psychiatry 1987; 150:782–6.

Guedeney N, Fermanian J, Guelfi JD, Kumar RC. The Edinburgh Postnatal Depression Scale (EPDS) and the detection of major depressive disorders in early postpartum: some concerns about false negatives. J Affect Disord 2000; 61(1–2):107–12.

Eberhard-Gran M, Eskild A, Tambs K, Opjordsmoen S, Samuelsen SO. Review of validation studies of the Edinburgh Postnatal Depression Scale. Acta Psychiatr Scand 2001; 104(4):243–9.

Dennis CL. Can we identify mothers at risk for postpartum depression in the immediate postpartum period using the Edinburgh Postnatal Depression Scale? J Affect Disord 2004; 78(2):163–9.

Address for correspondence

The Royal College of Psychiatrists
The British Journal of Psychiatry
17 Belgrave Square, London SW1X 8PG, UK
Telephone: +44 (0) 20 7235 2351
Email: publications@rcpsych.ac.uk

Edinburgh Postnatal Depression Scale (EPDS)

Instructions for users

1. The mother is asked to underline the response which comes closest to how she has been feeling in the previous 7 days.
2. All ten items must be completed.
3. Care should be taken to avoid the possibility of the mother discussing her answers with others.
4. The mother should complete the scale herself, unless she has limited English or has difficulty with reading.
5. The EPDS may be used at 6–8 weeks to screen postnatal women. The child health clinic, postnatal check-up or a home visit may provide suitable opportunities for its completion.

Name :

Address :

Baby's Age :

As you have recently had a baby, we would like to know how you are feeling. Please UNDERLINE the answer which comes closest to how you have felt IN THE PAST 7 DAYS, not just how you feel today.

1. I have been able to laugh and see the funny side of things.
   As much as I always could
   Not quite so much now
   Definitely not so much now
   Not at all

2. I have looked forward with enjoyment to things.
   As much as I ever did
   Rather less than I used to
   Definitely less than I used to
   Hardly at all

3. I have blamed myself unnecessarily when things went wrong.*
   Yes, most of the time
   Yes, some of the time
   Not very often
   No, never

4. I have been anxious or worried for no good reason.
   No, not at all
   Hardly ever
   Yes, sometimes
   Yes, very often

5. I have felt scared or panicky for no very good reason.*
   Yes, quite a lot
   Yes, sometimes
   No, not much
   No, not at all

6. Things have been getting on top of me.*
   Yes, most of the time I haven't been able to cope at all
   Yes, sometimes I haven't been coping as well as usual
   No, most of the time I have coped quite well
   No, I have been coping as well as ever

7. I have been so unhappy that I have had difficulty sleeping.*
   Yes, most of the time
   Yes, sometimes
   Not very often
   No, not at all

8. I have felt sad or miserable.*
   Yes, most of the time
   Yes, quite often
   Not very often
   No, not at all

9. I have been so unhappy that I have been crying.*
   Yes, most of the time
   Yes, quite often
   Only occasionally
   No, never

10. The thought of harming myself has occurred to me.*
    Yes, quite often
    Sometimes
    Hardly ever
    Never

Response categories are scored 0, 1, 2, and 3 according to increased severity of the symptoms. Items marked with an asterisk are reverse scored (i.e. 3, 2, 1, and 0). The total score is calculated by adding together the scores for each of the ten items. The EPDS may be photocopied by individual researchers or clinicians for their own use without seeking permission from the publishers. The scale must be copied in full and all copies must acknowledge the following source: Cox JL, Holden JM and Sagovsky R. Detection of postnatal depression. Development of the 10-item Edinburgh Postnatal Depression Scale. *Br J Psychiatry* 1987; 150: 782–86. Written permission must be obtained from the Royal College of Psychiatrists for copying and distribution to others or for republication (in print, online or by any other medium).

Geriatric Depression Scale (GDS)

Reference: **Yesavage JA, Brink TL, Rose TL, Lum O, Huang V, Adey M, Leirer VO. Development and validation of a geriatric depression screening scale: a preliminary report. J Psychiatr Res 1983; 17(1):37–49**

Rating Self-report

Administration time 20 minutes

Main purpose To assess depression in older adults

Population People aged over 65 years

Commentary

The GDS in its original format is a 30-item self-report questionnaire developed to assess depression over the past week in geriatric populations. An abbreviated 15-item version of the instrument (the GDS-15) that shows good correlation with the original scale is also in widespread use, and takes approximately 5 minutes to administer (Sheikh and Yesavage 1986). A number of even shorter versions of the GDS have also been developed (for example, Shah et al., 1997). The GDS utilizes a simple yes/no response format (to be administered either in writing or orally) and consists of brief, comprehensible items that purposefully omit somatic complaints. The scale is appropriate for use as a screening instrument for depression in geriatric populations and demonstrates good psychometric properties in terms of reliability and validity (it has been found to correlate well with both the Hamilton Depression Rating Scale, see page 28, and the Zung Self-Rating Depression Scale, see page 59). It is also seeing increasing use as an outcome measure.

Scoring

Items are scored in a yes/no (1/0) format with a total score range of 0–30 for the original version. Scores in the range of 0–1 are considered normal, 10–19 indicate mild depression, and 20–30 moderate to severe depression. A cut-off score of 9 shows 90% sensitivity and 80% specificity.

Versions

There are multiple translations of the GDS including: Chinese, Danish, Dutch, French, German, Greek, Hebrew, Hindi, Hungarian, Icelandic, Italian, Japanese, Korean, Lithuanian, Malay, Portuguese, Rumanian, Russian, Spanish, Swedish, Thai, Turkish, Vietnamese, and Yiddish. A 35-item clinician-administered version of the scale is also available.

Additional references

Sheikh JI, Yesavage JA. Geriatric Depression Scale (GDS): recent evidence and development of a shorter version. Clinical Gerontol 1986; 5:165–73.

Shah A, Herbert R, Lewis S, Mahendran R, Platt J, Bhattacharyya B. Screening for depression among acutely ill geriatric inpatients with a short Geriatric Depression Scale. Age Ageing 1997; 26(3):217–21.

Osborn DP, Fletcher AE, Smeeth L, Stirling S, Nunes M, Breeze E, Siu-Woon Ng E, Bulpitt CJ, Jones D, Tulloch A, Siu-Woon Ng Edmond. Geriatric Depression Scale Scores in a representative sample of 14 545 people aged 75 and over in the United Kingdom: results from the MRC Trial of Assessment and Management of Older People in the Community. Int J Geriatr Psychiatry 2002; 17(4):375–82.

Address for correspondence

Dr. Jerome Yesavage
Stanford University School of Medicine
Stanford, CA 94305-5548, USA
Telephone: 1-650-852-3287
Email: yesavage@stanford.edu
Website: http://www.stanford.edu/~yesavage/GDS.html

Geriatric Depression Scale (GDS)

1. Are you basically satisfied with your life?
2. Have you dropped many of your activities and interests?
3. Do you feel that your life is empty?
4. Do you often get bored?
5. Are you hopeful about the future?
6. Are you bothered by thoughts you can't get out of your head?
7. Are you in good spirits most of the time?
8. Are you afraid that something bad is going to happen to you?
9. Do you feel happy most of the time?
10. Do you often feel helpless?
11. Do you often get restless and fidgety?
12. Do you prefer to stay at home, rather than going out and doing new things?
13. Do you frequently worry about the future?
14. Do you feel you have more problems with memory than most?
15. Do you think it is wonderful to be alive now?
16. Do you often feel downhearted and blue?
17. Do you feel pretty worthless the way you are now
18. Do you worry a lot about the past?
19. Do you find life very exciting?
20. Is it hard for you to get started on new projects?
21. Do you feel full of energy?
22. Do you feel that your situation is hopeless?
23. Do you think that most people are better off than you are?
24. Do you frequently get upset over little things?
25. Do you frequently feel like crying?
26. Do you have trouble concentrating?
27. Do you enjoy getting up in the morning?
28. Do you prefer to avoid social gatherings?
29. Is it easy for you to make decisions?
30. Is your mind as clear as it used to be?

This is the original scoring for the scale: One point for each of these answers. Cutoff: normal 0–9; mild depressives 10–19; severe depressives 20–30.

1. no 6. yes 11. yes 16. yes 21. no 26. yes
2. yes 7. no 12. yes 17. yes 22. yes 27. no
3. yes 8. yes 13. yes 18. yes 23. yes 28. yes
4. yes 9. no 14. yes 19. no 24. yes 29. no
5. no 10. yes 15. no 20. yes 25. yes 30. no

Reproduced from Yesavage JA, Brink TL, Rose TL, et al. J Psychiatr Res 1983; 17(1):37–49.

Kutcher Adolescent Depression Scale (KADS)

Reference: **LeBlanc JC, Almudevar A, Brooks SJ, Kutcher S. Screening for adolescent depression: comparison of the Kutcher Adolescent Depression Scale with the Beck Depression Inventory. J Child Adolesc Psychopharmacol 2002; 12(2):113–26**

Rating Self-report

Administration time 3–5 minutes

Main purpose To screen for and assess the severity of adolescent depression

Population Adolescents

Commentary

The KADS is a recently developed 16-item self-report scale designed to identify adolescents with depression and to monitor symptom severity over time. A 6-item screening version of the scale is available, as well as an 11-item subscale optimized for sensitivity to change. Initial reports have indicated that the instrument shows good psychometric properties; a study of treatment outcome in adolescents diagnosed with major depression has demonstrated that the 11-item version is a sensitive measure of change in this population.

Scoring

Both self-report versions of the instrument are scored on a 0 to 3 scale. The 6-item scale yields a total possible score of 18, with scores ≥6 indicating possible depression, and a need for thorough diagnostic evaluation. The 11-item scale yields a total possible score of 33, with higher scores over time indicating worsening symptomatology, and lower scores suggesting improvement; there are no validated diagnostic categories associated with particular ranges of scores for this version.

Versions

No other versions are available.

Additional references

Brooks SJ, Krulewicz SP, Kutcher S. The Kutcher Adolescent Depression Scale: assessment of its evaluative properties over the course of an 8-week pediatric pharmacotherapy trial. J Child Adolesc Psychopharmacol. 2003;13(3):337–49.

Address for correspondence

Dr. Stanley Kutcher
5909 Veterans' Memorial Lane, Room 9209
QEII Health Sciences Centre, Lane Building
Halifax, Nova Scotia B3H 2E2, Canada
Telephone: 1-902-473-6214
Email: stan.kutcher@dal.ca

Kutcher Adolescent Depression Scale (KADS) – sample items

Over the last week, how have you been 'on average' or 'usually' regarding the following items:

1) low mood, sadness, feeling blah or down, depressed, just can't be bothered.
   a) hardly ever
   b) much of the time
   c) most of the time
   d) all of the time
2) feeling decreased interest in: hanging out with friends; being with your best friend; being with your spouse/boyfriend/girlfriend; going out of the house; doing school work or work; doing hobbies or sports or recreation.

   a) hardly ever
   b) much of the time
   c) most of the time
   d) all of the time
3) trouble concentrating, can't keep your mind on schoolwork or work, daydreaming when you should be working, hard to focus when reading, getting 'bored' with work or school.
   a) hardly ever
   b) much of the time
   c) most of the time
   d) all of the time

© 2002 Stan Kutcher

Kutcher Generalized Social Anxiety Disorder Scale for Adolescents (K-GSADS-A)

Reference: **Brooks SJ, Kutcher S. The Kutcher Generalized Social Anxiety Disorder Scale for Adolescents: Assessment of its evaluative properties over the course of a 16-week pediatric pharmacotherapy trial. J Child Adolesc Psychopharmacol 2004; 14:273–86**

Rating Clinician-rated

Administration time 20 minutes

Main purpose To assess the severity of social phobia and measure treatment outcome in adolescents

Population Adolescents aged 11–17 years

Commentary

The K-GSADS-A is a recently developed 29-item scale designed to assess baseline severity of social phobia in adolescents, and to monitor change in response to treatment intervention. Section A of the scale contains 18 items where, for each item, two ratings are made to index the patient's level of (i) discomfort/anxiety/distress associated with the situation, and (ii) avoidance of the situation. Section B prompts for up to 3 of the adolescent's most feared social situations; each of these situations is then rated for (i) fear and (ii) avoidance (note that on repeated administration of the K-GSADS-A, ratings would be made for the same situations specified at the initial assessment). Section C contains 11 items and assesses whether a particular treatment has differential effects on affective and somatic symptoms. Initial work has indicated that the scale shows sound psychometric properties (i.e. adequate internal consistency, good validity and good sensitivity to change) in adolescents with social phobia.

Scoring

Items in Sections A and B of the instrument are rated on a 4-point scale ranging from 0 (no discomfort/avoidance) to 3 (severe discomfort/total avoidance). Each item in Section C is rated for 'how strongly the symptom occurs in most social situations' on a scale of 0 (never experienced) to 3 (severe). The K-GSADS yields 4 sub-scales: (i) Fear and Anxiety (the sum of Section A's 18 discomfort ratings); (ii) Avoidance (the sum of Section A's 18 avoidance ratings); (iii) Affective Distress (the sum of Section C's 'affective' item scores); and (iv) Somatic Distress (the sum of Section C's 'somatic' item scores) and a total score (range 0–141): note that Section B items do not contribute to the total score.

Versions

No other versions are available.

Additional references

None available.

Address for correspondence

Dr. Stanley Kutcher
5909 Veterans' Memorial Lane, Room 9209
QEII Health Sciences Centre, Lane Building
Halifax, Nova Scotia B3H 2E2, Canada
Telephone: 1-902-473-6214
Email: stan.kutcher@dal.ca

Kutcher Generalized Social Anxiety Disorder Scale for Adolescents (K-GSADS-A) – sample items

Each item is rated for
(i)   the level of discomfort/distress/anxiety that the adolescent associates with the situation, and
(ii) the adolescent's level of avoidance of the situation on a scale of 0 (none) to 3 (severe/total avoidance)

- Feeling embarrassed or humiliated
- Experiencing a panic attack

In general, how strongly do these items occur to you in most social situations?
Scoring: 0 = Never; 1 = Mild; 2 = Moderate; 3 = Severe

- Attending a party or other social gathering with people you don't know very well
- Presenting in front of a small group or in a classroom setting
- Entering a classroom or social group once the class or activity is already underway

---

Multidimensional Anxiety Scale for Children (MASC)

Reference: **March JS. Manual for the Multidimensional Anxiety Scale for Children (MASC). 1997. Toronto, Canada, Multi-Health Systems**

Rating Self-report

Administration time 15 minutes

Main purpose To assess symptoms of anxiety in children and adolescents

Population Children and adolescents aged 8–19 years

Commentary

The MASC is a recently developed 39-item self-report measure designed to assess symptoms of anxiety in child and adolescent populations. The instrument assesses a wide array of anxiety symptoms (it covers all anxiety symptoms described in DSM-IV with the exception of those relating to OCD). The scale assesses 4 primary domains: physical symptoms (tense/restless and somatic/autonomic), social anxiety (humiliation/rejection and public performance fears), harm avoidance (perfectionism and anxious coping), and separation anxiety. Early results have indicated that the scale demonstrates good test–retest reliability (March and Sullivan, 1999). The MASC-10, a 10-item version, is designed for repeated testing and is a unidimensional measure that combines the 4 basic anxiety scales offered in the MASC. The MASC-10 takes about 5 minutes to administer and score and is recommended for group-testing situations. Both the original version of the scale and the MASC-10 demonstrate good ability to discriminate between children with anxiety disorders (with the exception of OCD) and healthy control subjects. Although not a diagnostic instrument per se, the scale is appropriate for use as part of a clinical diagnostic assessment.

Scoring

Items are scored on a 4-point scale (ranging from 1, never, though to 4, often) with a total score range of 39–156.

The scale provides a Total Anxiety score, an Anxiety Disorders Index and an Inconsistency Index.

Versions

The scale has been translated into: Afrikaans, Chinese, Canadian-French, Dutch, German, Hebrew, Italian, Lithuanian, Norwegian, Spanish, Swedish and Turkish.

Additional references

March JS, Parker JD, Sullivan K, Stallings P, Conners CK. The Multidimensional Anxiety Scale for Children (MASC): factor structure, reliability, and validity. J Am Acad Child Adolesc Psychiatry 1997; 36(4):554–65.

March JS, Sullivan K. Test–retest reliability of the Multidimensional Anxiety Scale for Children. J Anxiety Disord 1999; 13(4):349–58.

Compton SN, Nelson AH, March JS. Social phobia and separation anxiety symptoms in community and clinical samples of children and adolescents. J Am Acad Child Adolesc Psychiatry 2000; 39(8):1040–6.

Dierker LC, Albano AM, Clarke GN, Heimberg RG, Kendall PC, Merikangas KR, Lewinsohn PM, Offord DR, Kessler R, Kupfer DJ. Screening for anxiety and depression in early adolescence. J Am Acad Child Adolesc Psychiatry 2001; 40(8):929–36.

Address for correspondence

Multi-Health Systems Inc.
P.O. Box 950
North Tonawanda, NY 14120-0950, USA
Telephone: 1-800-456-3003 in the US
or 1-416-492-2627 international
Email: customerservice@mhs.com
Website: www.mhs.com

Revised Children's Manifest Anxiety Scales (RCMAS)

Reference: **Reynolds CR, Richmond BO. Revised Children's Manifest Anxiety Scale (RCMAS) Manual. 1985. Los Angeles, CA, Western Psychological Services**

Rating Self-report

Administration time 5 minutes

Main purpose To assess level and nature of anxiety in children and adolescents

Population Children and adolescents aged 5–19 years

Commentary

The RCMAS is a widely-used 37-item self-report questionnaire that constitutes a revision of the original Children's Manifest Anxiety Scale. The RCMAS is divided into 4 sub-scales: physiological anxiety, worry/over-sensitivity, social concerns/concentration, and a lie (social desirability) scale. A range of studies have now examined the psychometric properties of the instrument, which shows good reliability and validity (it correlates well with other measures of childhood anxiety). The scale is quick and easy to administer, either on an individual basis, or in a group setting. However, it is worth noting that the scale does not clearly correspond to DSM-IV anxiety disorder categories, and assesses a number of symptoms (i.e. mood, concentration, impulsivity) associated with other diagnoses.

Scoring

Items are scored in a yes/no format and the scale yields a 28-item Total Anxiety score (the remaining items constitute the lie scale) and 4 sub-scale scores.

Versions

The scale has been translated into French, German, Italian and Spanish.

Additional references

Reynolds CR, Richmond BO. What I think and feel: a revised measure of children's manifest anxiety. Abnorm Child Psychol 1978; 6(2):271–80.

Perrin S, Last CG. Do childhood anxiety measures measure anxiety? J Abnorm Child Psychol 1992; 20(6):567–78.

Address for correspondence

Western Psychological Services
12031 Wilshire Blvd.
Los Angeles, CA 90025-1251, USA
Telephone: 1-310-478-2061
Email: custsvc@wpspublish.com
Website: http://www.wpspublish.com

Revised Children's Manifest Anxiety Scales (RCMAS) – sample items

- I worry about what my parents will say to me

- It is hard for me to keep my mind on my schoolwork

Reynolds Adolescent Depression Scale, 2nd Edition (RADS-2)

Reference: **Reynolds WM. Reynolds Adolescent Depression Scale – Second Edition (RADS-2). In Hersen M (Series Ed.), Segal DL and Hilsenroth M (Vol. Eds.). Comprehensive Handbook of Psychological Assessment: Volume 2. Personality Assessment (pp. 224–236). 2004. New York, John Wiley & Sons**

Rating Self-report

Administration time 5–10 minutes

Main purpose To screen for depressive symptoms in adolescents

Population Adolescents aged 11–20 years

Commentary

The RADS-2 (a recently revised version of the original RADS) is a widely used 30-item self-report measure of depressive symptomatology for adolescents aged between 11 and 20 years. Respondents are requested to indicate how they usually feel, although the scale's items are worded in the present tense. The instrument is suitable for use as a screening instrument for depression in school-based or clinical settings, and there is some evidence that the instrument is sensitive to change in response to treatment. The instrument contains 4 sub-scales: dysphoric mood, anhedonia/negative affect, negative self-evaluation, and somatic complaints. A wide variety of studies have demonstrated that the original RADS showed good psychometric properties in a range of adolescent populations, including those with mental retardation, or emotional and behavioural problems. It also showed good correlation with both the Hamilton Depression Rating Scale (see page 28) and the Beck Depression Inventory (see page 10).

Scoring

Items are scored on a 4-point scale ranging from 1 (almost never) through to 4 (most of the time), with some reverse scoring. A total score (range 30–120, with higher scores indicating greater depression severity) for the scale is cal-culated by a simple sum of raw scores. Scoring can be completed by hand or computer. The manual suggests that a score of ≥77 may indicate clinical depression.

Versions

A 30-item version of the scale for children aged between 8 and 12 years (the Reynolds Child Depression Scale or RCDS) is also available. The RADS-2 has been translated into Hebrew and Spanish.

Additional references

King CA, Hovey JD, Brand E, Ghaziuddin N. Prediction of positive outcomes for adolescent psychiatric inpatients. J Am Acad Child Adolesc Psychiatry 1997; 36(10):1434–42.

Reynolds WM, Mazza JJ. Reliability and validity of the Reynolds Adolescent Depression Scale with young adolescents. J Sch Psychol 1998; 36(3):295–312.

Krefetz DG, Steer RA, Gulab NA, Beck AT. Convergent validity of the Beck depression inventory-II with the Reynolds adolescent depression scale in psychiatric inpatients. J Pers Assess 2002; 78(3):451–60.

Address for correspondence

Psychological Assessment Resources
16204 N. Florida Ave.
Lutz, FL 33549, USA
Telephone: 1-813-968-3003
Email: custserv@parinc.com
Website: www.parinc.com

Reynolds Adolescent Depression Scale, 2nd Edition (RADS-2) – sample items

- I feel lonely
- I feel upset

- I feel worried
- I feel happy

Worry Scale for Older Adults (WS)

Reference: Wisocki PA. Worry as a phenomenon relevant to the elderly. Behav Ther 1988; 19:369–79

Rating Self-report

Administration time 5–10 minutes

Main purpose To assess worry in older adults, specific to events commonly associated with aging

Population Older adults

Commentary

The WS is a 35-item self-report questionnaire designed to assess worry in older adults about social, financial and health issues. The instrument shows relatively sound psychometric properties; the scale's total score demonstrates good internal consistency in older adults with GAD (the instrument's sub-scales demonstrate slightly poorer internal consistency values) and fair test–retest reliability. An expanded 88-item version of the scale (WS-R) is also available that assesses 3 additional sub-scales: personal concerns, family concerns and world issues.

Scoring

Items are scored on a 0 (never) to 4 (much of the time, more than 2 times a day) scale. Total score range of the scale is 0–140, with higher scores indicating more frequent worry. Sub-scale scores are calculated by summing the appropriate items.

Versions

The scale has been translated into French, Hebrew and Spanish.

Additional references

Stanley M, Beck J, Zebb B. Psychometric properties of four anxiety measures in older adults. Behaviour Research and Therapy 1996; 34: 827–38.

Hunt S, Wisocki P, Yanko J. Worry and use of coping strategies among older and younger adults. J Anxiety Disord 2003; 17(5):547–60.

Address for correspondence

Dr. Patricia A. Wisocki
169 Browning Street
Wakefield, RI 02879, USA
Telephone: 1-401-789-1749
Email: wisocki@psych.umass.edu or
ptie389513@aol.com.

Worry Scale for Older Adults (WS)

INSTRUCTIONS: Below is a list of problems that often concern many Americans. Please read each one carefully. After you have done so, please fill in one of the spaces to the right with a check that describes HOW MUCH THAT PROBLEM WORRIES YOU. Make only one check mark for each item.

THINGS THAT WORRY ME ...

	Never	Rarely 1–2 times per month	Sometimes 1–2 times per week	Often 1–2 times per day	Much of the time More than 2 times a day
Finances					
1. I'll lose my home	☐	☐	☐	☐	☐
2. I won't be able to pay for the necessities of life (such as food, clothing, or medicine)	☐	☐	☐	☐	☐
3. I won't be able to support myself independently	☐	☐	☐	☐	☐
4. I won't be able to enjoy the 'good things' in life (such as travel, recreation, entertainment)	☐	☐	☐	☐	☐
5. I won't be able to help my children financially	☐	☐	☐	☐	☐
Health					
6. My eyesight or hearing will get worse	☐	☐	☐	☐	☐
7. I'll lose control of my bladder or kidneys	☐	☐	☐	☐	☐
8. I won't be able to remember important things	☐	☐	☐	☐	☐
9. I won't be able to get around by myself	☐	☐	☐	☐	☐
10. I won't be able to enjoy my food	☐	☐	☐	☐	☐
11. I'll have to be taken care of by my family	☐	☐	☐	☐	☐
12. I'll have to be taken care of by strangers	☐	☐	☐	☐	☐
13. I won't be able to take care of my spouse	☐	☐	☐	☐	☐
14. I'll have to go to a nursing home or hospital	☐	☐	☐	☐	☐
15. I won't be able to sleep at night	☐	☐	☐	☐	☐
16. I may have a serious illness or accident	☐	☐	☐	☐	☐
17. My spouse or a close family member may have a serious illness or accident	☐	☐	☐	☐	☐
18. I won't be able to enjoy sex	☐	☐	☐	☐	☐
19. My reflexes will slow down	☐	☐	☐	☐	☐
20. I won't be able to make decisions	☐	☐	☐	☐	☐
21. I won't be able to drive a car	☐	☐	☐	☐	☐
22. I'll have to use a mechanical aid (such as a hearing aid, bi-focals, a cane)	☐	☐	☐	☐	☐
Social Conditions					
23. That I'll look 'old'	☐	☐	☐	☐	☐
24. That people will think me unattractive	☐	☐	☐	☐	☐
25. That no one will want to be around me	☐	☐	☐	☐	☐
26. That no one will love me anymore	☐	☐	☐	☐	☐
27. That I'll be a burden to my loved ones	☐	☐	☐	☐	☐
28. That I won't be able to visit my family and friends	☐	☐	☐	☐	☐
29. That I may be attacked by muggers or robbers on the streets	☐	☐	☐	☐	☐
30. That my home may be broken into and vandalized	☐	☐	☐	☐	☐
31. That no one will come to my aid if I need it	☐	☐	☐	☐	☐
32. That my friends and family won't visit me	☐	☐	☐	☐	☐
33. That my friends and family will die	☐	☐	☐	☐	☐
34. That I'll get depressed	☐	☐	☐	☐	☐
35. That I'll have serious psychological problems	☐	☐	☐	☐	☐

Reproduced from Wisocki PA. Behav Ther 1988; 19:369–79. © Patricia Wisocki 1988.

Which scale to use and when

Assessment scales	Abbreviation	Self- or clinician- rated	Administration (minutes)
Depression – General			
Beck Depression Inventory – Second Edition	BDI-II	Self-report	5–10
Carroll Depression Scales–Revised	CDS-R	Self-report	20
Centre for Epidemiological Studies Depression Scale	CES-D	Self-report	10
Diagnostic Inventory for Depression	DID	Self-report	15–20
Hamilton Depression Inventory	HDI	Self-report	10–15
Hamilton Depression Rating Scale	HDRS, Ham-D	Clinician-rated	20–30
Hamilton Depression Rating Scale, 7-item version	Ham-D7	Clinician-rated	20–30
Harvard National Depression Screening Scale	HANDS	Self-report	10
Hospital Anxiety and Depression Scale	HADS	Self-report	<5
Inventory of Depressive Symptomatology	IDS	Self-report (IDS-SR) or Clinician-rated (IDS-C)	30–45
Montgomery–Asberg Depression Rating Scale	MADRS	Clinician-rated	5–10
MOS Depression Questionnaire	MOS-DQ	Self-report	<5
Patient Health Questionnaire 9	PHQ-9	Self-report	<5
Raskin Depression Rating Scale	RDRS	Clinician-rated	10–15
Zung Self-Rating Depression Scale	Zung SDS	Self-report (Zung SDS) or clinician-rated (Zung DSI)	5
Profile of Mood States	POMS	Self-report	<5
Depression – Subtypes			
BDI – FastScreen for Medical Patients	BDI-FS	Self-report	<5
Bech–Rafaelsen Melancholia Rating Scale	MES	Clinician-rated	10
Calgary Depression Scale for Schizophrenia	CDSS	Clinician-rated	20
Cornell Dysthymia Rating Scale	CDRS	Clinician-rated	20
Cornell Scale for Depression in Dementia	CSDD	Clinician-rated	30
Edinburgh Postnatal Depression Scale	EPDS	Self-report	5
Hamilton Depression Rating Scale, ADS version	SIGH-ADS	Clinician-rated	10–20
Hamilton Depression Rating Scale, SAD version	SIGH-SAD, Ham-SAD	Clinician-rated	10–20
Hospital Anxiety and Depression Scale (Medical patients)	HADS	Self-report	<5
Personal Inventory for Depression and SAD	PIDS	Self-report	15
Seasonal Pattern Assessment Questionnaire	SPAQ	Self-report	5–10
Suicide			
Beck Hopelessness Scale	BHS	Self-report	5–10
Beck Scale for Suicide Ideation	BSS	Self-report	5–10
Suicide Probability Scale	SPS	Self-report	5–10
Mania			
Bech–Rafaelsen Mania Scale	MAS	Clinician-rated	10
Clinician-Administered Rating Scale for Mania	CARS-M	Clinician-rated	15–30
Manic State Rating Scale	MSRS	Clinician-rated	15
Mood Disorders Questionnaire	MDQ	Self-report	5–10
Young Mania Rating Scale	YMRS	Clinician-rated	10–20
Anxiety – General			
Adult Manifest Anxiety Scale	AMAS	Self-report	10
Beck Anxiety Inventory	BAI	Self-report	5–10
Covi Anxiety Scale	COVI	Clinician-rated	5–10
Depression Anxiety Stress Scales	DASS	Self-report	10
Hospital Anxiety and Depression Scale	HADS	Self-report	<5
Penn State Worry Questionnaire	PSWQ	Self-report	5
State-Trait Anxiety Inventory (Form Y)	STAI	Self-report	20
Zung Self-Rating Anxiety Scale	SAS	Self-report	5

Population	Purpose	Rating sheet reproduced	Page
Adults and adolescents	To assess severity of depressive symptomatology	No	10
Adults	To assess severity of depressive symptoms	No	13
Adults and adolescents	To assess depressive symptomatology in the general population	Full scale	14
Adults	To diagnose depression according to DSM-IV criteria, and to assess psychosocial impairment and quality of life	Full scale	23
Adults	To provide a self-report version of the HDRS	Sample items only	27
Adults	To assess severity of, and change in, depressive symptoms	Full scale	28
Adults	To assess severity of, and change in, depressive symptoms	Full scale	30
Adults	To screen for major depressive disorder	Full scale	32
Adults and adolescents	To screen for depression and anxiety in medical patients	No	81
Adult inpatients or outpatients	To assess severity of, and change in, depressive symptoms	Full scale	33
Adults taking antidepressant medication	To assess depressive symptomatology, particularly change following treatment with antidepressant medication	Full scale	39
Adults under 60 years	To screen for depression and dysthymia	Full scale	37
Adults	To screen for depression in primary care	Full scale	49
Adult inpatients or outpatients	To assess severity of depressive symptoms, with a specific focus upon verbal report, behaviour and secondary symptoms	Full scale	50
Adults	To assess depressive symptomatology	Full scale	59
Adults	To assess mood state and changes in mood	No	148
Adults and adolescents	To screen for depression in medical patients	No	163
Adults and adolescents	To assess severity of depressive symptoms	Full scale	9
Adults and adolescents diagnosed with schizophrenia	To assess depressive symptoms separate from positive, negative and extrapyramidal symptoms in people with schizophrenia	Full scale	164
Adults and adolescents	To assess severity of symptoms of dysthymia	Full sccale	20
Patients with dementia	To assess depressive symptomatology in people with dementia	Full scale	169
Women who have recently given birth	To screen for postnatal depression	Full scale	172
Adults	To assess severity and change in depressive symptoms including atypical symptoms of depression	No	54
Adults	To assess severity of, and change in, depressive symptoms	No	55
Adults and adolescents	To screen for depression and anxiety in medical patients	No	82
Adults and adolescents	To screen for depression, seasonality in depressive symptoms and atypical neurovegetative symptoms	Full scale	46
Adults and adolescents	To screen for winter depression	Full scale	51
Adults and adolescents	To assess feelings of hopelessness about the future	No	11
Adults and adolescents	To assess severity of suicidal ideation	No	12
Adults and adolescents	To assess suicide risk	Sample items only	56
Adults and adolescents	To assess severity of symptoms of mania in patients with bipolar disorder	Full scale	8
Adults	To assess severity of manic and psychotic symptoms	Full scale	16
Adults	To assess severity of manic symptoms	Full scale	36
Adults	To screen for bipolar spectrum disorders	Full scale	42
Adults and adolescents with mania	To assess severity of manic symptoms	Full scale	57
Adults, college students and older adults	To assess the level and nature of anxiety in adults	Sample items only	65
Adults and adolescents	To assess symptoms of anxiety (particularly somatic)	No	69
Adults	To assess severity of symptoms of anxiety	Sample items only	72
Adults and adolescents	To detect core symptoms of depression, anxiety and stress using a dimensional approach	Full scale	75
Adults and adolescents	To screen for depression and anxiety in medical patients	No	82
Adults	To assess trait symptoms of pathological worry	Full scale	103
Adults, adolescents and children	To assess state and trait levels of anxiety	Sample items only	109
Adults	To measure symptoms of anxiety	Full scale	115

Assessment scales	Abbreviation	Self- or clinician- rated	Administration (minutes)
Anxiety – OCD			
Maudsley Obsessional Compulsive Inventory	MOCI	Self-report	5
Obsessive Compulsive Inventory	OCI	Self-report	15
Padua Inventory–Washington State University Revision	PI-WSUR	Self-report	10
Yale-Brown Obsessive Compulsive Scale	Y-BOCS	Clinician-administered	20–30 (less with repeat administrations)
Anxiety – Panic			
Anxiety Sensitivity Index	ASI	Self-report	<5
Anxiety Sensitivity Index–Revised 36	ASI-R-36	Self-report	5
Fear Questionnaire	FQ	Self-report	10
Panic and Agoraphobia Scale	PAS	Self-report or clinician-rated	5–10
Panic Disorder Severity Scale	PDSS	Clinician-rated	10
Mobility Inventory for Agoraphobia	MI	Self-report	10–20
Brief Social Phobia Scale	BSPS	Clinician-rated	5–15
Fear of Negative Evaluation Scale (FNE) and Social Avoidance and Distress Scale (SADS)	FNE, SADS	Self-report	10 each
Liebowitz Social Anxiety Scale	LSAS	Clinician-administered (LSAS-CA) and self-report (LSAS-SR)	20–30
Social Phobia and Anxiety Inventory	SPAI	Self-report	20–30
Social Phobia Inventory	SPIN	Self-report	10
Social Phobia Scale and Social Interaction Anxiety Scale	SPS & SIAS	Self-report	5 each
Anxiety – PTSD			
Clinician-Administered PTSD Scale	CAPS	Clinician-rated	45–60
Davidson Trauma Scale	DTS	Self-report	10
Impact of Event Scale-Revised	IES-R	Self-report	5–10
Posttraumatic Stress Diagnostic Scale	PDS	Self-report	10–15
Children/Adolescents			
Children's Depression Inventory	CDI	Self-report	10–15
Children's Depression Rating Scale, Revised	CDRS-R	Clinician or caregiver rated	15–20
Kutcher Adolescent Depression Scale	KADS	Self-report	3-5
Multidimensional Anxiety Scale for Children	MASC	Self-report	15
Kutcher Generalized Social Anxiety Disorder Scale for Adolescents	K-GSAD-A	Clinician-rated	20
Revised Children's Manifest Anxiety Scales	RCMAS	Self-report	5
Reynolds Adolescent Depression Scale, 2nd Edition	RADS-2	Self-report	5–10
Older Adults			
Cornell Scale for Depression in Dementia	CSDD	Clinician-rated	30
Geriatric Depression Scale	GDS	Self-report	20
Worry Scale	WS	Self-report	5–10
Other Symptoms			
Brief Pain Inventory	BPI	Self-report	5 (short form), 10 (long form)
Brief Psychiatric Rating Scale	BPRS	Clinician-rated	10–30
Brief Symptom Inventory	BSI	Self-report	10
Clinical Global Impression	CGI	Clinician-rated	Varies with familiarity with patient
Epworth Sleepiness Scale	ESS	Self-report	5
Fatigue Severity Scale	FSS	Self-report	5

Population	Purpose	Rating sheet reproduced	Page
Adults and adolescents	To assess obsessive-compulsive symptoms	Full scale	86
Adults	To assess severity of obsessive-compulsive symptoms	Full scale	90
Adults	To assess severity of obsessions and compulsions	Full scale	92
Adults	To measure severity of obsessive-compulsive symptoms	Full scale	110
Adults, adolescents and children	To measure anxiety sensitivity	No	65
Adults and adolescents	To assess anxiety sensitivity	Full scale	66
Adults	To measure severity of, and change in, common phobias and related anxiety and depression	Full scale	79
Adults	To assess severity of panic disorder (with or without agoraphobia)	Full scale	95
Adults	To assess severity of panic disorder	Full scale	99
Adults	To assess severity of agoraphobic avoidance and frequency of panic attacks	Full scale	88
Adults	To assess fear, avoidance and physiological arousal related to social phobia	Full scale	69
Adults	To assess fear of social evaluation and distress and avoidance in social situations	Full scale	76
Adults, adolescents and children	To measure fear and avoidance in patients with social phobia	Sample items only	84
Adults and adolescents	To assess symptoms of social phobia as defined by DSM-IV	No	105
Adults	To evaluate fear, avoidance and physical arousal in relation to social phobia	No	106
Adults	The SPS was developed to assess fear of being observed by others during routine activities, whereas the SIAS measures fear of social interaction	Full scale	107
Adults and adolescents	To diagnose and assess severity of PTSD	Sample items only	71
Adults	To assess symptoms of PTSD	No	73
Adults and adolescents	To assess distress (intrusion, avoidance and hyperarousal) associated with stressful life events	Full scale	82
Adults	To assess DSM-IV diagnostic criteria and symptom severity of PTSD	No	104
Children and adolescents aged 7–17 years	To assess depressive symptomatology	No	171
Children aged 6-12 and adolescents	To diagnose depression and assess treatment response in children	Sample items only	172
Adolescents	To diagnose and assess the severity of adolescent depression	Sample items only	181
Children and adolescents aged 8–19 years	To assess symptoms of anxiety in children and adolescents	No	183
Adolescents aged 11–17 years	To assess the severity of social phobia and measure treatment outcome in adolescents	Sample items only	182
Children and adolescents aged 5–19 years	To assess level and nature of anxiety in children and adolescents	Sample items only	184
Adolescents aged 11–20 years	To screen for depressive symptoms in adolescents	Sample items only	185
Patients with dementia	To assess depressive symptomatology in people with dementia	Full scale	174
People aged over 65 years	To assess depression in older adults	Full scale	179
Older adults	To assess worry in older adults, specific to events commonly associated with aging	Full scale	186
Adults	To assess the severity of pain and the impact of pain on daily functions	Full scale	120
Adults with psychiatric disorders	To assess psychiatric symptoms and severe psychopathology	Full scale	123
Adults and adolescents	To assess severity of psychological symptoms	No	125
Adults	To provide a global rating of illness severity, improvement and response to treatment	Full scale	126
Adults and older adults	To assess levels of daytime sleepiness	Full scale	131
Adults	To assess severity of fatigue	Full scale	136

Assessment scales	Abbreviation	Self- or clinician- rated	Administration (minutes)
General Health Questionnaire	GHQ	Self-report	Dependant on version
Pittsburgh Sleep Quality Index	PSQI	Self-report	5–10
Positive and Negative Syndrome Scale	PANSS	Clinician-rated	30–40
Primary Care Evaluation of Mental Disorders Patient Health Questionnaire	PHQ	Self-report	5
Short Form McGill Pain Questionnaire	SF-MPQ	Self-report	5
Somatic Symptom Inventory	SSI	Self-report	7
Symptom Checklist-90–Revised	SCL-90–R	Self-report	15
Side Effects			
Abnormal Involuntary Movement Scale	AIMS	Clinician-rated	5
Arizona Sexual Experiences Scale	ASEX	Self-report	5
Epworth Sleepiness Scale	ESS	Self-report	5
Extrapyramidal Symptom Rating Scale	ESRS	Self-report	15
Fatigue Severity Scale	FSS	Self-report	5
Pittsburgh Sleep Quality Index	PSQI	Self-report	5–10
Systematic Assessment for Treatment Emergent Events	SAFTEE	Clinician-rated	10–15
Somatic Symptom Inventory	SSI	Self-report	7
Functioning and Quality of Life			
Clinical Global Impression	CGI	Clinician-rated	Varies with familiarity with patient
Dartmouth COOP Functional Assessment Charts	COOP	Self-report	5
Duke Health Profile	DUKE	Self-report	5
Global Assessment of Functioning Scale	GAF	Clinician-rated	Very brief after patient evaluation
Medical Outcomes Study Short-Form 36	SF-36	Self-report	10
Quality of Life Enjoyment and Satisfaction Questionnaire	Q-LES-Q	Self-report	10
Sheehan Disability Scale	SDS	Self-report	<5
Sickness Impact Profile	SIP	Self-report	20+

Population	Purpose	Rating sheet reproduced	Page
Adults, adolescents and older adults	To screen for psychiatric distress related to physical illness	No	137
Adults, adolescents and older adults	To assess levels of daytime sleepiness and sleep disturbance	Full scale	141
Adults and adolescents	To assess severity of positive and negative symptoms in psychotic disorders	No	144
Adults	To assess mental disorders, functional impairment, and recent psychosocial stressors	Full scale	145
Adults, adolescents and older adults	To assess the sensory, affective and other qualitative components of pain	Full scale	154
Adults	To assess severity of somatic symptomatology	Full scale	164
Adults and adolescents	To screen for global psychopathology	No	166
Adults	To assess level of dyskinesias in patients taking neuroleptic medications	Full scale	116
Adults	To measure sexual functioning	Full scale (female version)	118
Adults and older adults	To assess levels of daytime sleepiness	Full scale	131
Adults, adolescents and children	To assess severity of extrapyramidal symptoms	Full scale	132
Adults	To assess severity of fatigue	Full scale	136
Adults, adolescents and older adults	To assess levels of daytime sleepiness and sleep disturbance	Full scale	141
Adults and adolescents	To detect and monitor treatment-emergent adverse events	Full scale	156
Adults	To assess severity of somatic symptomatology	Full scale	164
Varies with familiarity with patient	To provide a global rating of illness severity, improvement and response to treatment	Full scale	126
Adults and adolescents	To assess general health status and functioning	No	128
Adults	To assess general health status	Full scale	129
Adults	To measure global psychosocial functioning in psychiatric patients	Full scale	138
Adults	To assess perceived health status	No	140
Adults	To assess generic quality of life	Sample items only	150
Adults	To assess degree of disability	Full scale	152
Adults	To behaviourally assess the impact of sickness	No	163

Appendix 2

Alphabetic list of scales

Scale	Page